The Essential Oil Guidebook

CRAFTED BY SKRIUWER

Copyright © 2024 by Skriuwer.

All rights reserved. No part of this book may be used or reproduced in any form whatsoever without written permission except in the case of brief quotations in critical articles or reviews.

For more information, contact : **kontakt@skriuwer.com** (www.skriuwer.com)

TABLE OF CONTENTS

CHAPTER 1: INTRODUCTION TO ESSENTIAL OILS

- What They Are and Why They Matter
- Basic Terms and Common Uses
- Initial Safety Reminders

CHAPTER 2: THE HISTORY OF ESSENTIAL OILS

- Ancient Civilizations and Early Methods
- Middle Ages to Renaissance Developments
- Modern Refinements and Global Expansion

CHAPTER 3: FUNDAMENTAL CHEMISTRY OF ESSENTIAL OILS

- Main Chemical Components
- How Molecules Affect Aroma and Function
- Oxidation and Shelf Life

CHAPTER 4: PRODUCTION & EXTRACTION METHODS

- Steam Distillation, Cold Pressing, and More
- Solvent Extraction and CO2 Techniques
- Environmental Impacts and Quality Checks

CHAPTER 5: UNDERSTANDING QUALITY & PURITY

- Identifying Authentic Oils
- GC-MS Reports and Transparency
- Avoiding Adulteration and Marketing Traps

CHAPTER 6: SAFETY AND BEST PRACTICES

- Dilution Guidelines
- Phototoxic and Irritating Oils
- Safe Use Around Children, Elderly, and Pets

CHAPTER 7: ESSENTIAL OILS FOR STRESS AND RELAXATION

- Popular Calming Scents
- Methods: Diffusion, Inhalers, and Topical
- Combining Oils with Other Relaxation Techniques

CHAPTER 8: ESSENTIAL OILS FOR SLEEP & REST

- Common Oils for Better Nighttime Routines
- Blends and Practical Tips for Bedtime
- Supportive Habits Alongside Oils

CHAPTER 9: ESSENTIAL OILS FOR MOOD AND EMOTIONAL SUPPORT

- How Scent Affects Emotions
- Specific Oils for Different Moods
- Usage Ideas: Inhalers, Diffusers, and Topical

CHAPTER 10: ESSENTIAL OILS FOR SKIN & BEAUTY

- Skin Types and Matching Oils
- DIY Serums, Masks, and Infused Body Care
- Safety Steps to Avoid Irritation

CHAPTER 11: ESSENTIAL OILS FOR CHILDREN AND THE ELDERLY

- Special Dilution and Sensitive Skin Needs
- Preferred Oils for Different Age Groups
- Practical Tips and Warnings

CHAPTER 12: ESSENTIAL OILS IN HOUSEHOLD CLEANING

- *Natural Cleaning Ingredients*
- *Effective DIY Recipes*
- *Storage and Safety With Kids and Pets Around*

CHAPTER 13: ESSENTIAL OILS FOR FIRST AID AND COMMON HEALTH ISSUES

- *Minor Cuts, Burns, and Bug Bites*
- *Head Comfort and Muscle Support*
- *What to Do in Emergencies and When to Seek Help*

CHAPTER 14: ESSENTIAL OILS & AROMATHERAPY

- *Fundamental Principles and Methods*
- *Emotional Benefits and Relaxation*
- *Blending for Specific Goals*

CHAPTER 15: ESSENTIAL OILS IN CULINARY APPLICATIONS

- *Safe Oils for Cooking*
- *Recipes and Flavor Pairings*
- *Important Precautions and Correct Dosing*

CHAPTER 16: ADVANCED BLENDING TECHNIQUES

- *Aroma Families: Top, Middle, and Base Notes*
- *Crafting Complex, Balanced Blends*
- *Testing, Maturing, and Perfecting Formulas*

CHAPTER 17: ESSENTIAL OILS IN MASSAGE AND PHYSICAL THERAPY

- *Choosing Oils for Relaxation or Muscle Support*
- *Basic Massage Methods and Dilution*
- *Safe Use Within Physical Therapy Plans*

CHAPTER 18: ESSENTIAL OILS IN PET CARE

- *Risks and Caution for Cats, Dogs, and Other Pets*
- *Safe Diffusion Practices (If Any)*
- *Alternatives and Pet-Safe Recommendations*

CHAPTER 19: SETTING UP AN ESSENTIAL OIL BUSINESS

- *Business Models and Market Research*
- *Sourcing, Branding, and Legal Requirements*
- *Marketing, Distribution, and Long-Term Vision*

CHAPTER 20: FUTURE TRENDS AND ONGOING RESEARCH

- *Emerging Technologies and Sustainability Efforts*
- *Scientific Insights and Evolving Best Practices*
- *Projections for the Essential Oil Industry*

CHAPTER 1: Introduction to Essential Oils

1.1 What Are Essential Oils?

Essential oils are concentrated liquids taken from plants. These plants might be flowers, leaves, roots, or other parts. The liquids hold strong scents and helpful compounds that plants use to protect themselves. People have found ways to gather these fragrant liquids and use them for health, cleaning, and many other purposes.

Essential oils are called "essential" because they contain the "essence" or main scent of a plant. They are not oily in the same way cooking oils are. Instead, most essential oils feel thin and can evaporate quickly if left in open air. This quality is important and shows that these oils are made up of volatile compounds, which means they can move into the air and be smelled easily.

1.2 Why Essential Oils Matter

Essential oils have special qualities that have drawn human interest for many years. They can carry the scent of a plant and also contain substances that may support the body or mind. Each oil has a unique chemical makeup. This means some oils may help calm the mind, while others might clean surfaces well. A few might have strong smells that keep bugs away. There are also oils that can soothe mild skin irritations.

Today, people use essential oils for many reasons:

- Relaxation: Some scents, like lavender, may help with a calm mood.
- Focus: Citrus oils, like lemon, might make a room smell fresh and help with concentration.
- Skin care: Tea tree oil may help with mild skin problems.
- Cleaning: Oils like lemon, pine, or eucalyptus can add a fresh scent to home cleaning solutions.

1.3 Key Terms to Know

- **Volatile Compounds**: Chemicals that evaporate into the air and are easy to smell.
- **Diffusion**: A process of spreading the oil's scent through the air using a device or another method.
- **Carrier Oils**: Mild oils like fractionated coconut oil or sweet almond oil. These help dilute essential oils before they are applied to the skin.
- **Aromatherapy**: The practice of using scents, especially from essential oils, to improve well-being.

1.4 General Types of Essential Oils

There are many essential oils, and each falls into certain general scent groups. Some are citrus-like, such as lemon and orange. Others are herb-like, such as basil or rosemary. You can also find oils that come from trees and resins, like frankincense. Each type has different properties.

Here are some popular essential oils and their general uses:

- **Lavender**: Often linked with calmness.
- **Peppermint**: Popular for a cooling effect, often used for alertness.
- **Lemon**: Used for a fresh scent that may help lift the mood.
- **Tea Tree**: Valued for cleaning and skin applications.
- **Eucalyptus**: Known for a fresh scent that may help the airways feel clearer.

1.5 Benefits and Real-Life Uses

People often link essential oils with the mind. Some oils, when smelled, may help with calmer feelings or clearer thoughts. Others can be added to products like lotions or cleaning sprays. Certain oils have been studied for their antimicrobial qualities. For example, tea tree oil is sometimes added to foot care products. Lemon oil might be added to homemade disinfectants.

Real-life examples:

- **Adding Lavender Oil to a Bath**: A few drops in a bath can create a relaxing atmosphere.
- **Using Peppermint Oil on the Temples**: Some individuals find it helpful for mild head discomfort when diluted properly.
- **Making a Natural Room Spray**: A mixture of water, a small amount of rubbing alcohol, and a few drops of a citrus oil can make a fresh-smelling mist for rooms.

1.6 Basic Science Behind Essential Oils

Essential oils are complex. Each plant has many compounds in its oils. For example, lavender has linalool, which many believe is responsible for its calming scent. The chemistry of essential oils is important to understand because it helps us know which oils might be good for certain purposes. Some compounds are antibacterial. Others might have a pleasing scent that helps with easing tension.

1.7 Important Safety Notes

While these oils are natural, they are still very strong. A small bottle of essential oil may hold the compounds from many pounds of plant material. Because of this, it is wise to know how to handle them:

- **Dilution**: Always mix essential oils with a carrier oil before putting them on skin.
- **Patch Test**: Check how your skin reacts by testing a small amount of diluted oil.
- **Internal Use**: Do not ingest essential oils unless you have expert guidance. Many oils are not safe to eat.
- **Safety Around Pets and Children**: Some oils are not safe around animals or young children. Always store them in a safe place.

1.8 Simple Steps to Start Using Essential Oils

1. **Choose a Goal**: Do you want to make a room smell fresh? Do you want to use an oil in a foot bath?

2. **Pick the Right Oil**: Match the oil to the reason. For clearing the air, eucalyptus might be good. For a fresh scent in a kitchen, lemon might be useful.
3. **Use a Diffuser or a Simple Method**: An electric diffuser can spread the scent around. Or you can add a few drops to a bowl of steaming water.
4. **Consider Dilution if Using on Skin**: Mix a few drops of essential oil with a carrier oil.
5. **Watch for Reactions**: Stop use if any irritation or odd reaction occurs.

1.9 Myths About Essential Oils

Because these oils have been used for a long time, some myths have grown around them. Here are a few:

- **Myth: More is Better**: Using a lot of drops at once can cause irritation. Start with a small amount.
- **Myth: All Oils Are Safe for Everyone**: Not all oils are good for children, older people, or pets. Check guidance from a reliable source.
- **Myth: Essential Oils Can Replace All Medicines**: While they can help in some cases, they do not replace professional medical care.

1.10 Looking Ahead

In the following chapters, we will talk about how essential oils came into use, the science behind them, how to check for quality, and how you can safely mix them at home. We will also talk about some rare tips that might not be common knowledge, helping you get the most from these oils.

This first chapter gave a broad introduction. It should help you feel comfortable with the basic terms and ideas. The next chapter will go through how people in the past used these oils and how that shaped our current methods.

CHAPTER 2: The History of Essential Oils

2.1 Early Evidence of Plant Oils

Plants have been important to people since ancient times. Before there were modern labs, people still figured out how to press or steam plants to capture their fragrant materials. These early extracts might not have been as refined as modern essential oils, but they gave people a clue that plants held strong scents and could be used for practical reasons.

For example, ancient cultures around the world used certain scented resins in temples and during important events. These resins, when burned, would fill the air with distinct fragrances. Even before complicated distillation tools, people found simpler ways to extract scents by soaking plant material in fats or pressing flowers between layers of cloth.

2.2 Ancient Civilizations and Oils

Some of the earliest written records of scented plant extracts come from parts of Egypt and Mesopotamia. The Egyptians used fragrant substances for body care and also to help preserve bodies after death. Their methods included soaking or mixing plant parts with fats and then applying this mixture to hair and skin.

In ancient China, plant-based oils and extracts were used in early health practices. People recognized that different plants had different effects. Some seemed to help calm the mind, while others were used for minor aches.

In India, knowledge about oils appears in texts related to Ayurveda, a traditional system that dates back many centuries. These texts mention oils from plants like sandalwood, which was valued for its scent.

2.3 Distillation in Ancient Times

Distillation is a key step in creating essential oils. The ancient Persians are often credited with refining early distillation. Later, famous Arab scholars improved these techniques. One well-known figure was Avicenna (Ibn Sina).

He was not only a doctor but also an alchemist who studied ways to distill plants. Through methods involving heat and cooling, the vapors could be collected, and these vapors contained concentrated scents.

This method spread across the Middle East, Asia, and Europe. As trade routes grew, so did the exchange of knowledge about scents, plants, and ways to extract valuable materials. Distillation allowed people to produce more potent plant extracts.

2.4 The Use of Oils in Medieval Europe

By the Middle Ages, distillation had become more common in Europe. People used these extracts for many purposes, including attempts to ward off illness. Some mixtures included what we now know as thyme, rosemary, or clove oils. These plants have compounds that can help limit some types of microbes, though that was not fully understood back then.

Monasteries often had herbal gardens. Monks recorded information on plants and sometimes made simple herbal remedies. They might distill local plants to create small amounts of these scented extracts, which were then mixed into salves or used to mask unpleasant odors.

2.5 Growth in the Renaissance

During the Renaissance, exploration grew, and spices and plants from different parts of the world were traded widely. With more access to new plants, essential oil use grew. People became more aware that certain oils had specific effects. For example, oils from citrus fruit rinds, like bergamot or lemon, were brought back to Europe from foreign lands.

Apothecaries played a big role at this time. They sold herbs, spices, and plant-based preparations. Many apothecaries began to distill essential oils and experiment with new formulas. They labeled them as cures, mood enhancers, or ingredients for perfumes. This period set the stage for essential oils to be recognized both for their pleasant scents and potential health-related uses.

2.6 Modern Era and Essential Oils

With the invention of new technology during the Industrial Revolution, distillation methods became faster. Machines could heat large amounts of plant material. Innovations in glassmaking improved distillation equipment. This meant companies could produce bigger batches of essential oils, making them cheaper to buy.

In the early 20th century, interest in the scientific study of these oils grew. Researchers started isolating individual compounds, figuring out their chemical makeup. This gave the public and scientists a better grasp of why certain oils did what they did.

As the cosmetics and pharmaceutical industries expanded, they saw the value in using these plant-based materials. Perfume companies, for example, needed large amounts of flower oils to produce perfumes with consistent scents. This demand pushed more research on how to extract oils in a way that kept their scent strong.

2.7 How Aromatherapy Got Its Name

The term "aromatherapy" was first made known by a French chemist named René-Maurice Gattefossé in the 1920s. He studied how lavender oil seemed to help skin. His writings brought more attention to the idea that oils had special features beyond just smelling nice. Over time, more people started applying the term "aromatherapy" to describe the use of essential oils to support well-being.

Other figures in the mid-1900s promoted the use of oils and wrote books explaining the different effects of popular scents. By the 1970s, aromatherapy was gaining ground in places like the United States, the United Kingdom, and other parts of the world. Spas began offering treatments that used essential oils, and health food stores started stocking small bottles of different oils.

2.8 The Spread of Essential Oils Across the World

As global trade grew, so did the spread of essential oils. Plants once found only in certain regions were introduced to new places. For example, tea tree is native to Australia, but now tea tree oil is popular in many countries. Eucalyptus, which also comes from Australia, is now used around the world in rubs and inhalants to help clear the air.

Regions like France, Morocco, and Bulgaria are now known for their lavender fields. The flower is grown in large amounts to meet the global demand for lavender oil. On the other hand, places like Madagascar grow ylang-ylang, used in some luxurious perfumes and also known for a soft, floral scent.

2.9 Big Shifts in Quality and Regulation

As essential oils became more common, questions about quality and purity arose. Some sellers mixed oils with cheaper substances or synthetic fragrances. Others sold oils labeled with false claims. This led experts in various countries to call for stricter labeling rules.

Organizations formed to set guidelines for testing the contents of essential oils. These guidelines included checking chemical composition using scientific methods, such as gas chromatography. This testing helps ensure that what is in a bottle matches what is on the label.

2.10 Recent Trends in Essential Oils

In the last few decades, essential oils have grown in popularity among people who prefer more natural options. You might see oils in grocery stores, pharmacies, and online shops. They are added to soaps, shampoos, and even laundry products to give a plant-based aroma. Some companies also encourage their use for different kinds of home care or personal care.

However, along with rising use, there have been warnings from health experts about misuse. People sometimes use them without dilution or apply them to delicate skin areas. Others take them by mouth without checking for safety. These actions have led to more education on how to handle essential oils responsibly.

2.11 Cultural Contributions to Modern Knowledge

Over the centuries, various cultures have shared knowledge that still helps us today. Indigenous peoples often used local plants for wellness. Some had ways of extracting or preparing these plants that may resemble what we call essential oils. Their methods taught us about plants that can serve as bug repellents or that might soothe skin problems.

In the Middle East and parts of Asia, there was a long history of distillation that shaped modern methods. Even now, areas like India have large-scale production of essential oils from plants such as vetiver and patchouli. This global connection means that each region's unique plants and traditions feed into the world's overall knowledge about essential oils.

2.12 Lesser-Known Historical Facts

- **Distillation Apparatus in Ancient Civilizations**: While some credit the Persians for the first big steps in distillation, archaeological evidence suggests that other groups also did experiments with different forms of extraction.
- **Use of Fragrant Woods in Ceremonies**: Woods like cedar or sandalwood were burned during rites, and these were early forms of aromatherapy in a basic sense.
- **Essential Oils in the Spice Trade**: When traders traveled across oceans, they sometimes brought along materials like spice oils. These oils were easier to transport and sometimes used as currency or gifts.

2.13 The Impact of War and Travel

Wars and travel impacted the spread of essential oils, too. Soldiers and travelers might learn about local plants in new lands and bring home the knowledge. During World War I, there are records of essential oils being tested for cleaning wounds due to a shortage of supplies. While the results were mixed, this brought more attention to the possible use of these plant extracts.

Missionaries and explorers introduced plants from the Americas, Asia, and Africa to Europe. As these plants entered new markets, more people discovered their scents and benefits. Over time, gardens in Europe grew exotic plants like jasmine and geranium for the perfume trade.

2.14 Rise of Modern Brands and Marketing

In the 20th century, certain businesses began to market essential oils on a larger scale. They printed catalogs, showing how to use each oil, and also explained blends. This was when the idea of mixing oils to create special scent profiles became popular. Customers wanted to combine oils like lavender, rose, and sandalwood to get new aromas.

Some companies also put more money into research, working with universities to check the properties of certain oils. The marketing often pointed out not just the scent, but the potential ways it might help with stress or relaxation. Over time, direct selling businesses that focused on essential oils also appeared. They offered training, gave usage guides, and expanded the user base.

2.15 Important Milestones in Essential Oil History

- **Development of Modern Perfumes**: Starting in the 19th century, perfume houses in France used essential oils in large amounts. Advances in chemistry allowed them to isolate specific compounds that gave desired notes in fragrances.
- **Identification of Key Compounds**: Scientists started mapping out molecules like linalool, eugenol, or limonene. This helped match certain scents with the compounds responsible.
- **Growth of Aromatherapy Associations**: Groups of experts formed associations to share best practices, set professional standards, and encourage proper training.
- **Public Awareness Campaigns**: In the late 20th century, some health organizations began cautioning the public about unproven claims. This led to more balanced information about safe use of oils.

2.16 Challenges and Future Directions

Even with a long history, essential oils face challenges. One challenge is sustainability. Some plants are overharvested, leading to a risk that the natural environment might suffer. Another challenge is the spread of misinformation online, where claims can be made without evidence.

Despite these issues, many people remain interested in essential oils. They seek them out for adding pleasant scents to homes or for personal care. As the global market grows, more research is likely to uncover how these plant extracts can be used properly. We might see better technology for extraction and more details on how each oil interacts with the body and mind.

2.17 Summary of Historical Developments

1. **Ancient Use**: People in regions like Egypt, China, and India discovered the benefits of fragrant plants and started simple extraction methods.
2. **Improved Distillation**: The Middle East and later Europe refined distillation to produce more potent extracts.
3. **Expansion Through Trade**: The spice trade and exploration spread knowledge of different plant oils.
4. **Modern Growth**: The industrial era made distillation easier, while science explained the chemistry behind these scents.
5. **Aromatherapy Defined**: The term came into use in the 20th century, pushing essential oils into mainstream awareness.
6. **Global Acceptance**: Different regions now grow plants for essential oils, making them widely available.

2.18 A Look Ahead

The next chapters will cover the chemistry behind these oils, how they are made today, and how to pick the right type of oil for your needs. We will also look at topics like correct dosing, blending basics, and special uses. The historical background should help you see how these oils developed over time and why they are so widespread now.

Understanding their past can also help you avoid repeating past mistakes. In the history of essential oils, there were times people used them with little safety knowledge, and times when false claims were spread. Learning from those lessons can help you use these oils with more care today.

CHAPTER 3: Fundamental Chemistry of Essential Oils

3.1 Why Chemistry Matters

Chemistry is at the heart of what makes essential oils work. Each oil has a set of molecules that give it a distinct smell and possible effects. When you open a small bottle of oil, many different compounds rise into the air. These compounds travel through your nose to special cells that detect smells. Those signals then move to the brain, where they can influence how you feel. Some of these same molecules can also interact with skin when used in lotions or creams.

Understanding the chemistry of essential oils can help you decide which oil to use for a certain purpose. It also helps you store oils properly and blend them with more skill. Though the topic might seem difficult, we will keep it simple so you can still gather key points.

3.2 Basic Building Blocks: Molecules in Essential Oils

Essential oils are mainly made up of organic molecules. These molecules typically have carbon and hydrogen atoms, sometimes joined by oxygen atoms. Let's go over some common groups of molecules found in these oils:

1. **Terpenes**:
    - **Monoterpenes**: Common examples are limonene (found in citrus oils) and pinene (found in pine and some herbal oils). Monoterpenes usually have strong smells. They can evaporate quickly.
    - **Sesquiterpenes**: These are heavier compared to monoterpenes and do not evaporate as fast. An example is beta-caryophyllene, found in oils like clove and black pepper.
2. **Alcohols**:

- Some oils have alcohol-based molecules like linalool (found in lavender) or geraniol (found in rose). These can have gentler scents, and they often show mild effects on the skin.
3. **Phenols**:
   - Phenolic compounds can be more intense. Thymol in thyme oil is an example. These have potent properties and should be used carefully.
4. **Esters**:
   - Known for producing sweet or pleasant scents, esters include compounds like linalyl acetate, which is abundant in lavender. Esters are often linked with calming properties.
5. **Ketones and Aldehydes**:
   - These may have sharper smells. For instance, citronellal is an aldehyde found in citronella oil. Ketones and aldehydes should be used properly because some can irritate certain people.
6. **Oxides**:
   - One well-known oxide is 1,8-cineole (eucalyptol), commonly found in eucalyptus. It provides the recognizable scent that many link with clear breathing.

Each essential oil is a blend of many such molecules. The unique combination is why lemon oil smells fresh and bright, while rosemary oil has a strong, herb-like aroma.

3.3 How Molecules Affect Smell and Function

When you inhale an essential oil, your sense of smell picks up on the molecules that evaporate first. These are called top notes. Citrus oils and light herbal oils often have these top notes. As time passes, other molecules evaporate more slowly. They are called middle notes or base notes. Oils like patchouli or vetiver might have deeper notes that linger.

Each type of molecule may have different possible benefits. For example:

- **Monoterpenes**: May provide a fresh scent that can lift the atmosphere.

- **Sesquiterpenes**: Commonly found in grounding oils like cedarwood, which might be used for a sense of calm.
- **Esters**: Often mild and can be soothing for the skin when properly diluted.

It's helpful to remember that we do not need to memorize all molecule names, but knowing the general groups can guide us in choosing oils wisely.

3.4 Influence of Plant Parts and Growth Conditions

The chemistry of an essential oil can change based on:

- **Which part of the plant is used**: For example, bitter orange produces different oils from its peel (bitter orange oil), flowers (neroli), and leaves (petitgrain). Each of these oils has a distinct chemical composition.
- **Climate and Soil**: Plants grown in different regions might show changes in their main compounds. Lavender grown in high altitudes might have more linalool, while lavender grown in lower plains might show different levels of esters.
- **Harvest Time**: The time of day or stage of growth can affect the oil content in plants. Many farmers harvest at certain times when the compounds in the plant are at their peak.
- **Extraction Method**: The method used to pull out the oil can also change the final mix of molecules. Steam distillation may highlight certain compounds, while cold pressing for citrus peels might emphasize others.

These details show how complex each bottle of essential oil can be. That is also why different brands may smell slightly different even if they sell the "same" oil, like peppermint.

3.5 Synthetic vs. Natural Compounds

Many of the same molecules found in essential oils can be produced in labs. Perfume makers often use lab-made versions of natural scents to keep their fragrances consistent. While these lab-made molecules can smell almost the same, natural essential oils come with many different molecules mixed in, not just one or two.

For example, if you smell a pure rose essential oil, it may hold hundreds of minor components that give it a rich scent. A lab-made rose fragrance might include the main molecules that smell like rose, but it likely won't have every minor trace that can affect the overall feel.

This is one reason why some people prefer natural essential oils. They want the full range of plant compounds. Others might choose lab-made fragrances for cost reasons or to avoid variations. Either choice can have a place, but keep in mind that an essential oil's complete chemical fingerprint is what sets it apart from a synthetic fragrance.

3.6 Oxidation and Rancidity

Because essential oils have many compounds that can react with air, storing them the right way is key. Over time, exposure to oxygen, heat, or light can cause the molecules in the oil to change. This process is known as oxidation. When oxidation happens, the oil might smell different or become irritating to the skin.

Steps to reduce oxidation:

- **Tighten Caps**: Keep the bottle closed firmly when you are not using it.
- **Dark Glass Bottles**: Many oils come in amber or cobalt blue bottles to limit light exposure.
- **Cool Storage**: A shelf away from direct sunlight or a refrigerator can help slow oxidation.
- **Smell Test**: If the oil smells sharp or "off," it might have oxidized.

Once an oil is oxidized, it can be more likely to irritate the skin, so it's wise to discard it. Some oils oxidize more quickly than others. Citrus oils are known to have a shorter shelf life, around one to two years. Heavier oils like patchouli or sandalwood can last longer.

3.7 Chemistry and Blending

The science of blending essential oils relies on an understanding of their molecules. If you combine two oils that both have a high amount of monoterpenes, you might get a fresh but short-lasting aroma. If you add a base note oil with sesquiterpenes, the scent might gain depth and stay longer in the air.

When blending, many people follow a rule of combining top, middle, and base notes. This approach can create a balanced aroma that unfolds in layers. For example:

- **Top Note**: Lemon or bergamot for a bright first impression.
- **Middle Note**: Lavender or rosemary that forms the main character of the scent.
- **Base Note**: Cedarwood or patchouli to add depth and longevity.

While this is a simplified view, it helps beginners create pleasant blends. As you gain more experience, you might choose to keep track of the chemical families you're mixing. That way, you can aim for certain effects or scents by understanding the chemistry behind each oil.

3.8 Rare Facts: Lesser-Known Chemical Insights

1. **Chiral Molecules**: Some compounds in essential oils have mirrored forms. The way these forms show up in an oil can affect how we smell them.
2. **Synergy**: Certain oils might have a stronger effect together than they do alone. This is called synergy, and it can happen when molecules from different oils boost each other's effects.

3. **Seasonal Variations**: A plant harvested in the wet season may have different chemical strengths compared to the dry season. This can be seen in oils from certain herbs or flowers where rainfall patterns change their growth.
4. **Influence of Altitude**: High-altitude plants can have more stress from the environment, leading them to produce certain compounds in bigger amounts. This can alter the final essential oil chemistry.

These less obvious details can interest people who want to know how the environment shapes an oil's final profile.

3.9 Common Misconceptions About Essential Oil Chemistry

- **Misconception: Essential Oils Are Simple**: In fact, they contain hundreds of compounds. Each one can affect the overall aroma and potential effects.
- **Misconception: One Main Molecule Is Everything**: While a key molecule might define the oil's main scent, the minor ones can still shape how it works.
- **Misconception: All Oils Are Equally Safe**: Some oils are higher in certain compounds that can irritate the skin if not diluted. It's important to know the chemistry before use.
- **Misconception: Heating Oils Ruins Them Instantly**: Mild warming, like in a diffuser, will not completely ruin the oil, but very high temperatures over a long time can change the chemistry.

3.10 Practical Tips for Chemistry-Conscious Use

1. **Check the GC-MS Report**: Some reliable brands provide a Gas Chromatography-Mass Spectrometry report. This shows the key compounds in each batch. It can help confirm quality.
2. **Learn Basic Terms**: Knowing if an oil is high in monoterpenes (like limonene) or esters (like linalyl acetate) can guide your usage.

3. **Store with Care**: Chemistry is affected by heat, light, and air. Follow proper storage to keep your oils fresh.
4. **Dilute Properly**: The concentration of certain compounds can be strong. Diluting reduces the chance of irritation and can help the oil's scent layers stand out better.

3.11 Summary

Essential oil chemistry is not just for scientists in labs. A simple grasp of the main chemical groups can improve your ability to pick and use these oils. Knowing that each oil has a range of molecules allows you to respect its power. This knowledge also helps you handle the oil in a safe way. In short, chemistry is the map that helps explain why certain oils smell or behave a certain way.

Understanding that each compound works differently also helps you see why no two essential oils are exactly the same. This variety is what makes them fun to explore. By embracing basic chemistry principles, you can confidently bring essential oils into your daily life.

CHAPTER 4: Production and Extraction Methods

4.1 Why Extraction Matters

Essential oils come from parts of plants like leaves, flowers, bark, roots, and fruit peels. How we extract those oils can greatly affect their smell, color, and overall quality. Some methods use heat. Others use mechanical force. Certain oils require special approaches to preserve their delicate chemicals.

When you buy an essential oil, it is helpful to know how it was made. Different processes can yield oils with slightly different aromas or chemical profiles. For example, steam-distilled lime oil smells different from cold-pressed lime oil.

4.2 Steam Distillation

Steam distillation is one of the most popular methods to produce essential oils. This process involves:

1. **Heating Water**: A still (a large pot or container) with water is heated until it produces steam.
2. **Passing Steam Through Plant Material**: The plant material sits above the water. As steam moves through it, tiny oil droplets are released.
3. **Cooling and Separating**: The steam carrying the oil molecules travels into a cooling system. This changes the vapor back to liquid form, separating water from oil.

The essential oil, which does not mix easily with water, floats on top or sometimes sinks, depending on its density. Then it is carefully collected. Steam distillation works well for many plants, including lavender, peppermint, and rosemary. It is efficient and does not require chemicals, though the heat can sometimes break down delicate compounds.

4.3 Hydro Distillation

Hydro distillation is closely related to steam distillation. The main difference is that the plant material is soaked in water rather than suspended above it. As the water is heated and turns to steam, it draws the oil out of the plant. This method can be used for materials like rose petals or certain barks.

Some producers prefer hydro distillation for flowers that might be too delicate for regular steam distillation. However, soaking can sometimes lead to more water-soluble compounds mixing in. This might create variations in the final fragrance.

4.4 Cold Pressing (Expression)

For citrus fruits like lemon, orange, and bergamot, a different method is often used: cold pressing. In ancient times, people would manually squeeze or press the peels to release the aromatic oils. Today, machines can do this on a large scale:

1. **Washing and Grating**: Citrus rinds are lightly grated or pierced to help release the oil.
2. **Pressing**: The fruit is pressed, and the liquid that comes out has both juice and oil.
3. **Centrifugation**: A machine spins the mixture at high speed to separate the oil from the juice.

Cold pressing does not use heat, so the resulting oil smells close to the fresh peel. However, these oils may have a shorter shelf life because they can contain bits of wax or other elements from the peel. This method is also limited mostly to citrus fruits.

4.5 Solvent Extraction

Some plants produce very little essential oil or have oils that are easily damaged by heat. In these cases, producers might use solvents, like hexane or ethanol, to pull out aromatic compounds. There are a few steps:

1. **Soaking in Solvent**: Plant material is combined with a solvent that dissolves the aromatic molecules.
2. **Filtration**: The solid parts of the plant are removed, leaving a mixture of solvent and fragrant compounds.
3. **Solvent Removal**: By changing the temperature or pressure, the solvent is removed, leaving behind a concentrate called a concrete or an absolute (depending on the steps).

Concretes are waxy solids with a strong smell. To create an **absolute**, the concrete is further processed with alcohol. The alcohol extracts the aroma compounds, and once the alcohol evaporates, you get an absolute. Absolutes are typically used in perfumery because of their intense fragrance. However, traces of solvents can remain, so some people might avoid these products for personal care.

4.6 CO2 Extraction

A more modern method uses carbon dioxide (CO_2) under high pressure and low temperatures. In this process:

1. **Pressurized Chamber**: CO_2 is turned into a fluid under supercritical conditions (high pressure and a temperature above its critical point).
2. **Passing Through Plant Material**: The fluid CO_2 acts like a solvent, pulling out aromatic compounds.
3. **Releasing Pressure**: When pressure is released, the CO_2 goes back to a gas, leaving behind the extracted oil.

This method can yield extracts that closely resemble the original plant aroma. Also, there is no leftover chemical solvent, which is appealing to many who want a more "clean" method. CO_2 extraction works well for certain plants that might be challenging with steam distillation. However, it can be more expensive due to specialized equipment.

4.7 Enfleurage (Historic Method)

Enfleurage is an old technique that was once popular for extracting scents from delicate flowers like jasmine or tuberose. It is rarely used on a large scale today, but it offers insight into historical perfume-making. The process is:

1. **Fat Sheets**: Spread a layer of fat (like lard) on a glass plate.
2. **Flower Petals**: Place fresh petals on the fat. Over time, the fat absorbs the scent.
3. **Replacing Petals**: Remove old petals and replace them with fresh ones to increase the fragrance strength.
4. **Extracting the Oil from Fat**: The fat, now saturated with fragrance, is called pomade. To get the aromatic compounds out, the pomade is washed with alcohol.

Enfleurage was a slow and labor-intensive process, so modern methods have largely replaced it. Yet it remains a fascinating part of the history of fragrance extraction.

4.8 Maceration

Maceration is another older technique. Plant material is soaked in hot oil (often a carrier oil) to draw out its scent and beneficial compounds. The mixture is then strained. The result is not technically an "essential oil" but rather an infused oil. People sometimes do this at home with herbs like calendula or chamomile for skin care. While it doesn't produce a pure essential oil, it's a simple way to harness some plant properties.

4.9 Distillation Times and Fractions

During steam distillation, different chemical fractions may be released at different times. For example:

- **Top Fraction**: Some volatile molecules come out first, giving a bright smell.

- **Middle Fraction**: The bulk of the aromatic compounds may collect during the main distillation period.
- **Late Fraction**: Heavier or more heat-resistant compounds might come out later.

Some producers may collect these fractions separately to control the final aroma. Others combine everything into one batch. Shorter distillation times might capture lighter notes, while longer distillation might pull out deeper ones. These decisions can affect how an oil smells and what it can be used for.

4.10 Quality Control and Adulteration

Unfortunately, not all producers are honest about how they make oils. Some may dilute their products with cheaper oils or synthetic scents. This is why it's good to buy from a reputable company. The following points can help with quality control:

1. **Transparency**: Trustworthy brands often share which extraction method they use.
2. **Testing**: Gas Chromatography-Mass Spectrometry (GC-MS) test results can help confirm purity.
3. **Price Check**: If an oil is suspiciously cheap, it might be watered down or mixed with synthetic ingredients.
4. **Labeling**: Look for the botanical name. If a label only says "pure lavender oil" without a Latin name like *Lavandula angustifolia*, it might be questionable.

Knowing how an oil is extracted and that it has passed quality checks is key for safe and effective use.

4.11 Environmental Impacts

Extraction can put a strain on the environment if done recklessly. Some concerns include:

- **Deforestation**: Certain trees, like sandalwood, are heavily harvested.
- **Overharvesting Wild Plants**: Wild plant populations may diminish if not sustainably managed.
- **Energy Use**: Steam distillation and CO2 extraction can use significant energy, which can lead to a larger carbon footprint.
- **Chemical Pollution**: Solvent extraction can be risky if the chemicals are not handled or disposed of properly.

Choosing oils from suppliers who focus on sustainable farming or fair-trade practices can help reduce negative impacts.

4.12 Large-Scale vs. Small-Scale Production

Large-scale producers use industrial machinery that can process huge amounts of plant material. They aim to create consistent batches of oil for global markets. Small-scale producers might focus on niche or specialty oils, using small stills or CO2 extraction units. The final product may be pricier but can have a distinctive aroma due to careful handling.

Some people prefer small-batch oils for their unique profiles. Others rely on large brands for cost and consistency. Both approaches have value. It often comes down to personal preference and budget.

4.13 Unique Extraction Methods for Special Plants

1. **Resin Tapping**: For oils like frankincense or myrrh, the resin is collected from cuts in the bark. This resin is then steam-distilled to obtain the oil.
2. **Floral Waters**: When rose or other flowers are steam-distilled, the leftover water is called a hydrosol. It contains small amounts of the oil's compounds and is sometimes used for gentle skin toners.
3. **Fractional Distillation**: In some cases, the distillation can be done in stages under varied pressures to isolate specific compounds. This can produce very refined oils aimed at the perfume industry.

4.14 Key Points When Selecting Oils Based on Extraction

- **Heat-Sensitive Plant**: If you know a flower is very delicate, it might be better to look for a solvent or CO2-extracted product rather than steam-distilled.
- **Budget**: Absolutes and CO2 extracts can be more expensive. Steam-distilled oils are often more affordable.
- **Application**: For direct skin use (with proper dilution), some people prefer steam-distilled or cold-pressed oils. For crafting perfumes, absolutes or CO2 extracts might offer a richer scent.
- **Scent Profile**: Cold-pressed citrus oils usually smell very fresh, but a steam-distilled citrus oil might smell a bit softer or more subtle.

4.15 Simple Home Extraction Methods

While industrial extraction requires special tools, you can try a few methods at home:

1. **Basic Steam Distillation Setup**: A pot with water, a rack for plant material, and a way to collect the condensed steam.
2. **Infused Oil**: If you want to extract mild properties, place chopped herbs in a carrier oil and warm them gently on low heat for a period.
3. **Powdering and Soaking**: Some people grind spices and soak them in alcohol, then strain for a lightly scented extract (not a pure essential oil, but can still be fragrant).

These basic methods won't give you the same quality or concentration as commercial-grade essential oils, but they can be fun for experimentation.

4.16 Myths About Extraction

- **Myth: Cold-Pressed Is Always Better**: Cold-pressed works well for citrus rinds, but it's not the only "best" method. Each plant has an ideal approach.

- **Myth: All Solvent Extracts Are Unsafe**: While some might contain traces of solvent, reputable brands can produce safe absolutes for perfumery or limited skin application.
- **Myth: Homemade Distillation Always Yields Perfect Oil**: Home setups can be inconsistent. Professional equipment is designed to optimize yield and quality.

4.17 Special Focus: Yield and Plant Material

One reason essential oils can be expensive is the large amount of plant material needed. For instance:

- **Rose Oil**: Thousands of rose petals might be needed to produce a small amount of oil.
- **Jasmine Absolute**: Fresh jasmine flowers must be processed quickly, often at night or early morning, to capture their aroma.
- **Lemon Oil**: Even though the rind is more plentiful, you still need many lemons to get a small quantity of cold-pressed oil.

High yields can bring costs down, while low yields from scarce materials can drive up the price. This also reflects the effort and resources needed to grow, harvest, and process plants into oil.

4.18 Ensuring Longevity of Extracted Oils

After the extraction is complete, the producer must store the oils properly. Large barrels made of stainless steel or glass are common. The environment should be free from temperature extremes. Humidity and sunlight can also degrade the oils.

Once the oils leave the factory, they go to different points of sale. Bottling must be done carefully. If you see an oil in a clear plastic bottle, that might not be ideal. Dark glass helps protect the oil. Over time, even well-stored oils can change, so it's important to check recommended shelf life.

4.19 Putting It All Together

Extraction methods vary, and each choice affects the oil's final makeup. Here is a quick rundown:

- **Steam Distillation**: Great for many herbs, flowers, and seeds. Common and cost-effective.
- **Cold Pressing**: Mainly for citrus rinds; preserves a bright aroma.
- **Solvent Extraction**: Used for delicate flowers or plants that do not yield enough oil through distillation; results in concretes and absolutes.
- **CO2 Extraction**: A modern approach that keeps more of the plant's original aroma; can be pricier.
- **Enfleurage/Maceration**: Rarely used on a commercial scale today, but historically interesting.

By understanding these methods, you can better assess the product you are buying. This knowledge helps you choose oils that align with your preferences, whether you want a certain scent or a more "natural" process.

4.20 Conclusion

Production and extraction lie at the core of essential oil quality. Each step, from picking the plant at the right time to packaging the final oil, plays a role in how good (or not so good) the oil is. Techniques like steam distillation are tried and tested, while modern approaches like CO2 extraction offer new ways to capture complex scents.

As you move forward, being aware of these methods can help you pick top-notch oils. You can also avoid misleading or adulterated products by looking for information on how the oil is made. The next part of this book will explore how to check quality and purity, along with how to use these oils safely. That way, you can enjoy the best of what nature's aromatic liquids have to offer, without risks or worries.

CHAPTER 5: Understanding Quality and Purity

5.1 Why Quality Matters

When buying essential oils, we want the product to match what is on the label. Since essential oils come from plants, many factors can affect the final bottle. Poor handling, mixing with cheap fillers, or using old plant material can affect how an oil smells and works.

Quality and purity are linked. A pure oil should contain only the natural substances that come from the plant. If someone adds other materials, it is no longer pure. In this chapter, we will learn how to spot a quality product and why it is worth getting oils from good sources.

5.2 Common Marketing Terms

Many companies use terms like "therapeutic grade" or "clinical grade." These terms are not regulated by a single global authority. They can mean different things for different brands. This can confuse people who are trying to compare products.

1. **Therapeutic Grade**: Often a marketing term to suggest high quality. But there is no official group that gives out a "therapeutic grade" stamp.
2. **Food Grade**: Some essential oils may be labeled as safe to add to foods, but this depends on local rules. Even if an oil is labeled safe for cooking, it does not always mean it is right for every user.
3. **Pure**: A label that claims "100% pure" should mean the oil has no additives or synthetic chemicals. But not all sellers stick to this honestly.

Because these words are not always backed by law, it is wise to dig deeper before buying. We will see how to do this soon.

5.3 Methods to Check Quality

A few methods can help us figure out if an essential oil is high quality:

1. **GC-MS Testing**: Gas Chromatography-Mass Spectrometry is a scientific test. It shows which compounds are in an oil and in what amounts. A trustworthy seller may offer GC-MS reports or let you see them on request.
2. **Organoleptic Testing**: This is a fancy term for using your senses (smell, sight) to judge an oil. An experienced person can often tell if an oil is off by its scent or color.
3. **Physical Checks**: Some producers measure density or the optical rotation of an oil to confirm purity.

A single test might not say everything, but together they paint a good picture. If a brand claims high standards but will not share any test results, that is a warning sign.

5.4 Labels and Botanical Names

A proper label is another sign of quality. Look for:

- **Common Name**: For example, "Lavender Oil."
- **Botanical Name**: For lavender, it might be *Lavandula angustifolia* (sometimes written as *Lavandula officinalis* or *Lavandula vera*).
- **Part of Plant**: Some labels note if the oil comes from leaves, flowers, bark, or roots.
- **Extraction Method**: For instance, "Steam Distilled" or "Cold Pressed."
- **Country of Origin**: This can be important if you want an oil from a specific region known for that plant.
- **Batch or Lot Number**: Helps track the oil if there is a question about purity later.

If a label only says "lavender oil" without a botanical name or origin, it might not be the real variety you want. There are many types of lavender.

Some smell more herbal, and some are more floral. Without knowing the exact type, you do not know what you are buying.

5.5 Synthetic Additions and Adulteration

Sometimes sellers mix real essential oil with cheaper synthetic scents or carrier oils. This helps them save money, but it misleads buyers who expect a genuine product. Adulteration can happen in many ways:

1. **Adding Synthetic Fragrance**: A few drops of something that smells like lavender can fool the nose if you are not familiar with the real oil.
2. **Mixing Cheaper Oils**: Blending a low-cost oil with a pricier one.
3. **Stretching with Carrier Oils**: Mixing a real essential oil with a carrier oil like soybean oil, then labeling the bottle as pure essential oil.

In some cases, these mixtures can reduce the oil's potential benefits. They might also lead to skin irritation if the synthetic part is not skin-friendly. This is why it is important to know how to spot a reliable brand.

5.6 Organic vs. Non-Organic

You might see labels claiming "organic." This typically means the plants were grown without certain pesticides or chemical fertilizers. Organic essential oils can be a good choice if you are trying to avoid residues from farm chemicals. However, organic certification often costs money, and smaller farms might skip it even if they follow eco-friendly practices.

If you prefer organic, check if the label has a credible certification logo. You can also research the farm or supplier. Some small producers are not certified but follow natural growing methods. Others might have partial organic practices. In the end, the chemical tests can still matter more than a label alone.

5.7 Price and Availability

Price can sometimes hint at quality, but it is not the only factor. A pure rose oil, for example, is very expensive because it takes a lot of petals to make a small amount of oil. If you see "rose oil" for a very low price, be wary. It might be diluted or synthetic.

Some oils are naturally cheaper. Citrus oils often cost less because the rinds are more readily available, and cold pressing is easier. When comparing prices, look at the average market range for that specific oil. If the price is much lower than normal, that is a red flag. If it is much higher, it might just be the seller marking up the product, or it might be a special variety.

5.8 Shelf Life and Freshness

Essential oils do not last forever, especially those high in monoterpenes, like citrus oils. After some months or a couple of years, the oil can oxidize and smell stale. Heavier oils, like patchouli and vetiver, can last longer.

Ask the seller about the distillation or pressing date if possible. If the oil has been sitting on a shelf for years, its smell and potency might have changed. Storing an oil in a cool, dark place can help it last longer. But eventually, it will still degrade.

5.9 Choosing a Trustworthy Seller

A trustworthy seller is open about:

- **Source**: Where the plants come from and how they are grown.
- **Extraction Method**: Whether it is steam-distilled, cold-pressed, or something else.

- **Testing**: Sharing or at least talking about GC-MS or other quality checks.
- **Proper Labeling**: Giving you the botanical name, lot number, and best-before date.

They should also respond to questions in a clear way. If a company does not know the answers or tries to avoid them, consider looking elsewhere.

5.10 At-Home Tests and Simple Checks

While professional tests are best, there are a few simple checks you can try at home:

1. **Blot Test**: Put one drop of the oil on white paper. Real essential oils (except for some very thick ones) tend to evaporate without leaving a greasy stain. If it leaves an oily ring, it might be mixed with a carrier oil.
2. **Smell Over Time**: Pure oils often change scent notes as they evaporate. Synthetic mixtures might smell overly simple or remain the same from start to finish.
3. **Compare Bottles**: If you have two bottles of the same oil from different brands, compare their smell. They should be somewhat similar, though small differences are normal. If one smells too "fake" or overly strong, it might be suspect.

Keep in mind these are basic checks, not foolproof tests. But they might help you spot a very poor product.

5.11 Importance of Batch Consistency

Plants grow differently each season, so each distillation batch can vary. A high-quality brand might note these differences. Some big companies blend oils from different batches to create a uniform aroma year after year. Others might sell each batch as-is, so buyers experience natural variations.

There is no "right" or "wrong" here. Some people like consistency, especially if they use an oil in products they sell. Others enjoy the seasonal changes in scent that come from nature. Either way, consistency in testing and labeling is what matters.

5.12 Rare Facts on Purity Issues

- **White Oils**: Some oils, like frankincense, can be bleached or redistilled to remove color or strong smells. This might be done for cosmetic reasons, but it changes the natural makeup of the oil.
- **Recombined Oils**: Some companies separate certain molecules from an oil, then put some back in to tweak the scent. They might still label it as "pure," though it has been altered in a lab.
- **Essential Oil vs. Extract**: If something is labeled "extract," it might have used solvents or other processes that are different from standard distillation.

These hidden details show that "pure" is not always as straightforward as it sounds. Being an informed buyer helps you avoid surprises.

5.13 Reading Ingredient Lists in Blends

Sometimes you might buy a blend of oils (like a pre-mixed "sleep blend"). Check if the label lists all the oils used. A good brand will list each oil (such as lavender, chamomile, and sandalwood) in descending order of quantity. If a blend includes a carrier oil, it should also be listed.

Some blends do not disclose exact ratios because it is a "proprietary formula." Still, they should give you a general idea of what is inside and whether there are synthetic elements. Avoid blends that hide everything behind words like "fragrance" or "essence."

5.14 Use of GC-MS Reports

A GC-MS report shows a chart with peaks. Each peak represents a compound in the oil. A skilled chemist can read it to confirm if the oil's makeup matches what you expect. For instance, if you see a major peak for linalool and linalyl acetate in a lavender oil, that is a good sign. If the report shows odd peaks for synthetic chemicals, that suggests adulteration.

Some companies post these reports online. Others might email them if you ask. While most casual users may not read them in detail, the willingness to provide them can show that a seller takes purity seriously.

5.15 Personal Sensitivity and Preferences

Even if an oil is pure, some people might be sensitive to its smell or effects. Quality does not always mean it is right for you. For example, a pure cinnamon bark oil is strong. It can irritate skin if not diluted properly. A pure peppermint oil can feel intense and might cause discomfort for individuals with certain sensitivities.

If you have had negative reactions in the past, you may prefer oils that are gentler or ones that have gone through a partial redistillation to remove harsh compounds. Always test a small amount on your skin (in a carrier oil) to see how you respond.

5.16 Ethical and Sustainable Practices

Pure quality also involves ethical sourcing. Some plants, like sandalwood or rosewood, are at risk due to overharvesting. A good brand will ensure sustainable methods, like replanting and fair wages. They might have certifications or statements about these efforts.

Sustainability can also mean working with farmers who use responsible water and land management. This helps protect the environment while still producing the plants we need for oils. If you care about these issues, look for brands that mention them and can back up their claims with proof.

5.17 Storage and Handling at Home

Even the best oil can degrade if stored poorly. At home, follow these tips:

1. **Dark Glass Bottles**: Keep the oil in its original bottle or another dark glass container.
2. **Cool, Dry Place**: Heat and humidity speed up oxidation. A cabinet away from direct sunlight is good.
3. **Tight Caps**: Oxygen breaks down the oil. Close the bottle firmly after each use.
4. **Avoid Contamination**: Do not pour leftover oil back into the bottle if it touched another surface or was mixed with other substances.

By keeping your oils in good shape, you can enjoy their scents and properties for a longer time.

5.18 Helpful Questions to Ask Sellers

1. "Do you test each batch of oil for purity? If so, which tests do you use?"
2. "Can I see or request the GC-MS report for this oil?"
3. "Where is this oil sourced from?"
4. "Are there any additives or carrier oils mixed in?"
5. "Does this product have a best-before date?"

A knowledgeable seller should be able to answer without avoiding the topic. If they react poorly to these questions, that is a clue you might want to buy elsewhere.

5.19 Special Insights on Rare Oils

When dealing with rarer oils like Melissa (lemon balm) or Helichrysum, you might see very high prices. These plants produce less oil, so the cost is understandable. Be especially cautious if you see a rare oil at a bargain price. Some unscrupulous vendors may pass off blends of cheaper oils or synthetics as rare ones.

For instance, pure Melissa oil has a unique lemony smell with herbal hints. Some sellers might substitute lemon and citronella to mimic that. Checking GC-MS results or buying from a trusted brand is vital for these special oils.

5.20 Conclusion

Quality and purity can make a big difference in how well essential oils serve you. By looking at labels, checking for tests, and being alert to suspiciously low prices, you can avoid poor products. A trustworthy seller will be open about their sourcing and testing, and they will label their oils in a clear way.

When you invest in high-quality essential oils, you can feel more certain that the product aligns with what you expect. The next chapter will cover safety guidelines. Having pure oils is important, but using them the right way is also key. By knowing both quality factors and good practices, you can enjoy these oils without worries.

CHAPTER 6: Safety and Best Practices

6.1 Why Safety Is Essential

Essential oils come from natural sources, but they can still cause harm if used the wrong way. A single drop can contain the compounds of many plants. This concentrated power is why people value them. It is also why we must handle them with care.

In this chapter, we will see how to use essential oils in a safe way. This includes diluting them, knowing which oils to avoid in certain situations, and preventing accidents at home.

6.2 General Dilution Guidelines

Most skin problems happen when someone applies oils "neat," meaning undiluted. While a few oils might be safe to dab directly on the skin in tiny amounts (like some forms of lavender for short-term use), it is safer to dilute all oils.

- **Adults**: A common dilution range is about 1% to 3% for everyday use. This means 1 to 3 drops of essential oil per teaspoon (5 mL) of carrier oil.
- **Children**: For young kids, many experts recommend about 0.25% to 0.5% dilution (1 drop in 4 teaspoons of carrier oil). Babies under three months often should not use most essential oils at all, unless under expert advice.
- **Special Cases**: Some oils like clove or cinnamon bark are very strong and may need even lower dilution. If you are not sure, go with the lowest dilution first.

Carrier oils can be coconut, jojoba, sweet almond, or others. The idea is to spread out the essential oil molecules so they are less likely to irritate the skin.

6.3 Patch Testing

Before using a new oil on a larger area of skin, do a patch test:

1. **Dilute the Oil**: Follow the guidelines above.
2. **Apply to a Small Spot**: The inside of the forearm is a common spot.
3. **Wait 24 Hours**: Watch for redness, itching, or bumps.
4. **Stop If There Is a Problem**: If you see a reaction, wash with mild soap and water, and do not use that oil on your skin again.

This simple step helps avoid major reactions, especially if you have sensitive skin or allergies.

6.4 Phototoxicity

Certain citrus oils can cause the skin to be extra sensitive to sunlight or tanning beds. This is called phototoxicity. Oils like bergamot, lime, and lemon can contain furanocoumarins, which lead to skin burns or discoloration when exposed to UV light.

- **Check Labels**: Some bergamot or lime oils are labeled "furanocoumarin-free," meaning they have removed the risky compounds.
- **Wait Time**: If you use a phototoxic oil on your skin, you might need to avoid direct sun on that area for up to 12 or even 24 hours.
- **Dilution**: Lowering the concentration can also reduce the risk, but it's often best to avoid using these oils on skin if you plan to be in sunlight.

6.5 Ingestion: Yes or No?

Some sellers suggest putting essential oils in water or taking them in capsules. Others warn against it. The truth is, essential oils are very strong, and ingesting them can harm your digestive tract or organs if you do not have proper guidance. Many experts say avoid internal use unless a qualified professional (like a doctor or a certified clinical aromatherapist) says it is safe.

Common concerns with ingestion:

- **Irritation**: Oils can burn or irritate the throat, stomach, or mouth.
- **Toxicity**: Some oils are toxic if taken in large amounts, such as wintergreen (high in methyl salicylate).
- **Drug Interactions**: Oils might affect how medicines are absorbed.

If you are set on ingestion, do thorough research and consult a professional. But for most people, using essential oils on the skin or in a diffuser is enough.

6.6 Safe Diffusion Guidelines

Diffusing oils into the air is popular for changing the mood of a room or for breathing support. But there are still safety measures:

1. **Duration**: Diffuse for about 15–30 minutes at a time, then take a break. Running a diffuser all day might be too much for some people.
2. **Ventilation**: Keep a window slightly open or ensure the room is not sealed shut. This helps prevent overwhelming the space with fragrance.
3. **Amount**: Start with a few drops. You can add more if needed.
4. **Audience**: If you have visitors, make sure they do not have sensitivities or allergies. Pets can also be affected.
5. **Children**: Use a lesser amount around kids, and ensure the room is not too small or closed off.

Diffusion can be a gentle way to enjoy oils if you do it with care.

6.7 Using Essential Oils Around Babies, Kids, and the Elderly

Children and older adults often have thinner or more delicate skin. Their systems might also be more responsive to strong substances. Some points to keep in mind:

- **Age Restrictions**: Many experts advise no essential oils for newborns unless your medical professional approves.
- **Safe Oils Only**: For a toddler, mild oils like lavender or chamomile might be acceptable (in low dilution). Hot oils like oregano or cinnamon are often discouraged.
- **Short Sessions**: Limit the time of diffusion. Check if the child or older adult is comfortable.
- **Check Medications**: The elderly might be on medicines. Some oils could interact with them. Always consult a healthcare provider if you are unsure.

A small patch test or a short diffusion is often enough to see if there is any negative reaction.

6.8 Pregnancy and Nursing Considerations

Pregnancy is a special time, and certain essential oils might not be advised. While research is limited, caution is wise. Some oils are known to stimulate blood flow or have strong actions that might cause concerns.

- **First Trimester**: Many professionals advise avoiding most essential oils to reduce any risks, unless a qualified practitioner says otherwise.
- **Later Stages**: Some mild oils may be acceptable at low dilutions. Lavender or a small amount of citrus oil might be fine for room fragrance, but check with your healthcare provider.
- **Nursing**: Oils can pass through skin contact and possibly affect the baby. Again, seek professional advice for safe usage.

When in doubt, it is often best to skip or greatly reduce essential oil use during pregnancy and nursing unless you have expert guidance.

6.9 Hot Oils and Skin Sensitivity

Some oils are called "hot" because they can irritate or burn the skin if not diluted enough. These often include:

- Oregano
- Cinnamon Bark
- Clove
- Thyme (certain types)

If you want to use them, keep the dilution level very low (like under 1%). It might be wise to choose gentler oils for everyday needs. If you have sensitive skin, testing small amounts is key.

6.10 Essential Oils and Pets

Pets have different physiology from humans. Some oils can be harmful to them, especially to cats. Cats lack certain enzymes that help break down compounds in essential oils. Exposure to some oils (like tea tree or citrus) can cause problems for them.

- **Diffuser Caution**: If you diffuse oils, make sure your pet can leave the room. Avoid strong or long diffusion times.
- **Topical Use**: Be careful when applying essential oils to a dog or cat. Their sense of smell is stronger than ours, and they might lick the oils off.
- **Birds**: Birds can be very sensitive to fumes. Diffuse with care if you have birds in the home.

It is best to speak with a vet who knows about essential oils if you want to use them around animals.

6.11 Possible Drug Interactions

Some essential oils could interact with medications, either by amplifying their effects or reducing them. For example:

- **Blood Thinners**: Oils rich in eugenol (like clove) might have mild blood-thinning effects.
- **Blood Pressure Drugs**: Some oils that affect circulation might not mix well with certain medicines.
- **Sedatives**: Oils with calming effects, like lavender, could add to the sedative effect of medication.

If you are on regular meds, consult a healthcare provider to avoid any unwanted interactions. This is especially important for older adults or those with chronic conditions.

6.12 Handling Emergencies

If someone has a bad reaction to an essential oil:

1. **Skin Irritation**: Rinse the area with mild soap and water. You can also apply a carrier oil to the irritated spot, which may help dilute and reduce the effect of the essential oil.
2. **Eye Contact**: Rinse with cool water for several minutes. Seek medical help if stinging continues.
3. **Ingestion Accident**: Do not make the person vomit. Call a poison control center or go to the emergency room right away.
4. **Breathing Troubles**: Move to fresh air. If severe, get medical help.

Store oils in places where children and pets cannot reach them. Keep a clear label on each bottle.

6.13 Allergies and Sensitivities

Some people are allergic to certain plants or plant families. For instance, if you are allergic to ragweed, you might also react to chamomile oil because it belongs to a related plant group. Always be cautious when trying a new oil for the first time.

Symptoms of an allergic reaction may include:

- Redness or rash
- Itching
- Hives
- Trouble breathing in severe cases (seek help if this happens)

Stop use right away if you suspect an allergy.

6.14 Best Practices for Daily Use

1. **Keep It Simple**: Start with a small collection of oils you trust. Learn how each one affects you before you expand.
2. **Use a Carrier**: Whether applying to skin or making a roller blend, always include a carrier oil.
3. **Rotate Oils**: Some experts suggest not using the same oil in large amounts every day to lower the chance of sensitization (developing a skin reaction over time).
4. **Track Usage**: Write down which oils you have used and any reactions. This can help you spot patterns.

6.15 Possible Hormone Effects

Some people worry that certain oils might affect hormones. For example, lavender and tea tree have been studied for a possible link to hormone disruption. The evidence is not conclusive, but it is good to know about these discussions. If you have hormone-related concerns, reduce or avoid these oils until you talk with a healthcare provider.

6.16 Using Oils in Public Spaces

If you want to bring essential oils to the office or a group area, remember that not everyone enjoys or tolerates the same scents. Some people have asthma or migraines triggered by fragrances.

- **Ask First**: Check if coworkers or friends are okay with oils in the room.
- **Go Light**: Use fewer drops in the diffuser.
- **Ventilate**: Keep windows open if possible.

Being respectful of others' space is part of safe and responsible use.

6.17 Rare Tips for Extra Caution

- **Label Your Blends**: When you mix oils, label the bottle with the name and date. This avoids confusion later.
- **Keep a Reference Book or Chart**: Having a simple chart with maximum dilutions for children or pregnancy can prevent mistakes.
- **Do Not Store in Plastic**: Over time, essential oils can break down certain plastics, potentially contaminating the oil and damaging the container.
- **Avoid Ears and Eyes**: Never drip oils directly into the ears or near the eyes. These areas are very sensitive.

These tips can reduce accidents and keep usage organized.

6.18 Setting Up a Safe Blending Area

If you plan to blend oils at home:

1. **Clean Surface**: Wipe down counters to avoid mixing leftover drops from past blends.
2. **Well Ventilated Room**: This helps if you spill something or a strong odor makes you lightheaded.

3. **Gloves and Glassware**: Wear gloves if you handle strong oils or large amounts. Use glass or stainless steel tools that can be cleaned well.
4. **Proper Storage**: Keep your finished blends in labeled glass bottles with tight caps.

A little organization goes a long way toward safe blending and measuring.

6.19 Listening to Your Body

Each person's reaction to a scent or oil can be different. If you feel dizzy, nauseated, or uneasy from an oil, stop using it. Not every oil is suited for everyone. Some people can handle strong oils, while others get headaches from the same scent.

This is why it helps to do short test periods. Try diffusing an oil for 10 minutes. Check how you feel. If all is well, you can gradually increase the time next time. The goal is to build a safe and pleasant experience, not to rush.

6.20 Conclusion

Safety with essential oils is about respecting their power. We have learned about dilution, patch testing, and common pitfalls. We have also covered special concerns for pets, children, pregnant women, and older adults. By following these tips, you can enjoy the scents and potential benefits of essential oils while lowering the chance of harm.

Always remember, if you are unsure, ask a qualified professional. Essential oils are helpful tools when used the right way. They can add fresh aromas to a home, help with simple wellness tasks, or boost a relaxing setting. But they need careful handling to avoid problems.

In the chapters ahead, we will look at essential oils for stress relief, better rest, and emotional support, and we will explore how to add them to your daily routines wisely. Having a strong safety foundation will make those topics more practical and easier to apply.

CHAPTER 7: Essential Oils for Stress and Relaxation

7.1 Introduction to Stress

Stress is a common part of life. It can show up when you face changes, deadlines, or unexpected events. A bit of stress can sometimes help you act quickly. But too much stress can affect your mind and body in a negative way. You might feel tension in your muscles, notice changes in your mood, or have trouble focusing.

People look for ways to handle stress so it does not get out of control. Some prefer exercise or meditation, while others might speak with a counselor. Essential oils can also be added to a stress-management plan. They are not a cure for major problems, but they can play a small part in helping you find calm.

7.2 The Mind-Body Connection

The human brain and body work together. When stress shows up, your body releases certain hormones, like cortisol, which prepare you to handle a challenge. If stress is short-term, things often go back to normal. But in long-term stress, these hormones stay active, which might lead to problems like sleep troubles, high blood pressure, or anxious thoughts.

Scent can have a powerful effect on how we feel because our sense of smell is directly linked to parts of the brain that control mood. This is why certain aromas might help ease tension, while others might give you a small lift of energy. Essential oils tap into this mind-body link by sending smell signals that may calm the brain.

7.3 Common Causes of Stress

- **Work Pressure**: Tight deadlines, meetings, or high expectations.
- **Family or Relationship Issues**: Arguments, worrying about loved ones, or a busy household.

- **Health Problems**: Dealing with chronic illness or recovering from injuries.
- **Financial Concerns**: Bills, debt, or job security.
- **Change or Uncertainty**: Moving to a new place, changing jobs, or facing unknown outcomes.

Recognizing where stress comes from is the first step to handling it. Then you can pick methods—like essential oils—that help in a gentle, supportive way.

7.4 Why Essential Oils Can Help

When you smell an essential oil, the small smell particles travel through your nose to a special area in your brain. This region handles emotions, memory, and moods. Some oils have components that might lower feelings of tension or may guide the body to feel calmer.

Using these oils in diffusers, personal inhalers, or diluted on the skin might help create a sense of ease. Remember, they do not fix all problems. But they can be a handy tool when combined with healthy habits. Some people also find the act of choosing an oil and inhaling it to be a soothing ritual in itself.

7.5 Popular Stress-Reducing Oils

Many essential oils have calming qualities, but a few stand out:

1. **Lavender (Lavandula angustifolia)**
    - Known for a gentle, floral aroma.
    - Often linked to calm feelings.
    - Can be diffused, applied (diluted) on the wrists, or added to bathwater.
2. **Roman Chamomile (Chamaemelum nobile)**
    - Has a sweet, apple-like scent.
    - Often used for soothing the mind.
    - Works well at bedtime or in a calming blend.
3. **Bergamot (Citrus bergamia)**
    - A citrus oil with a light, fresh smell.
    - Some find it helpful for easing tension.

- o Must be used with care in the sun because it can cause phototoxicity unless it is a special type with fewer problem compounds.
4. **Sweet Orange (Citrus sinensis)**
    - o Bright, fruity scent that many people find uplifting.
    - o May help shift mood to a more positive state.
    - o Good for diffusers in shared spaces.
5. **Cedarwood (Cedrus atlantica or Juniperus virginiana)**
    - o Woody, grounding aroma.
    - o May help quiet racing thoughts.
    - o Often combined with floral oils to create a balanced blend.
6. **Ylang Ylang (Cananga odorata)**
    - o Strong, sweet, floral scent.
    - o Some find it comforting, but it can be intense, so using less is often better.

Each person's sense of smell is different. One oil might work well for one person but not for another. You can try different aromas to see which makes you feel at ease.

7.6 Methods to Use Essential Oils for Relaxation

1. **Diffusion**
    - o Use an electric diffuser or a candle-based one.
    - o Add 3–6 drops of your chosen oil to the water.
    - o Let it run for 15–30 minutes, then turn it off to avoid overwhelming the room.
2. **Personal Inhaler**
    - o A small tube with a cotton wick inside.
    - o Place 5–10 drops of essential oil on the wick.
    - o Close the tube and inhale when stress hits, or carry it in your pocket.
3. **Topical Application**
    - o Mix 1–3 drops in a teaspoon of carrier oil (like sweet almond or jojoba).
    - o Apply to wrists, neck, or shoulders.
    - o Breathe in the aroma as you rub it gently on your skin.
4. **Bath Soak**

- Add 5–8 drops to a tablespoon of carrier oil or liquid soap, then stir into a warm bath.
- Enjoy the soothing scent as you soak for 15 minutes or more.

5. **Room Sprays**
    - Mix about 10–15 drops of essential oil in 1 ounce of water or witch hazel.
    - Shake well and spray in the air.
    - Test first to avoid staining surfaces or furniture.

7.7 Rare Tips for Stress Management with Oils

- **Rotating Oils**: If you use lavender every day, you might get used to it. Switch to chamomile or cedarwood now and then for fresh results.
- **Pairing Aromas with Activities**: If you light a diffuser when you start a calming activity (like journaling), your brain can link that aroma with a relaxed feeling. This might help your mind settle faster the next time you smell that oil.
- **Combining Citrus and Floral**: Blending a citrus oil, like sweet orange, with a floral oil, like lavender, can balance an aroma that is too sweet or too sharp on its own.
- **Small Pocket Bottles**: Keep a tiny bottle of diluted oil in your bag. Take a sniff when you start to feel tense.
- **Diffusing at Work**: If allowed, use gentle oils like sweet orange or bergamot in a small diffuser at your desk. Check with coworkers in case of sensitivities.

7.8 Using Essential Oils Alongside Other Methods

Essential oils work best if you support them with healthy habits:

- **Breathing Exercises**: Inhale slowly, hold for a moment, and exhale softly. This can improve the effect of calming oils.
- **Stretching**: Release muscle tension by doing simple stretches, especially around the shoulders and neck.
- **Journaling**: Writing down your thoughts can clear your mind of racing ideas.

- **Relaxing Music**: Play soft music while diffusing oils to create a more serene space.

By combining essential oils with methods like these, you might notice a bigger impact than using oils alone.

7.9 Mistakes to Avoid

1. **Overusing Strong Oils**: Oils like ylang ylang or patchouli can be quite intense. A few drops might be enough.
2. **Ignoring Allergies**: Do a patch test or a small smell test before using a new oil.
3. **Using Too Many Oils at Once**: Blending too many can become overwhelming or result in a muddy scent.
4. **Relying Only on Oils**: If your stress is severe, talk to a professional. Essential oils are just one part of a larger plan.

7.10 Calming Blends to Try

1. **Gentle Floral Mix**
    - Lavender: 3 drops
    - Roman Chamomile: 2 drops
    - Cedarwood: 1 drop
    - Use in a diffuser with water.
2. **Bright Citrus Lift**
    - Bergamot: 2 drops
    - Sweet Orange: 3 drops
    - Geranium (optional): 1 drop
    - Diffuse or make a room spray with 1 ounce of witch hazel.
3. **Grounding Woody Blend**
    - Cedarwood: 3 drops
    - Frankincense: 2 drops
    - Mandarin: 2 drops
    - Diffuse in the evening after a busy day.

Feel free to tweak the number of drops based on your preference. If the aroma feels too strong, reduce the drops.

7.11 Monitoring Results

Pay attention to how you feel before and after using an essential oil. Maybe keep a small diary noting which oil you used, the method of use, and how you felt an hour later. Over time, you may notice a pattern. Perhaps lavender consistently helps you unwind, while sweet orange gives you a more sunny outlook. This feedback can guide future choices.

7.12 When to Seek Further Help

Essential oils can help ease mild stress, but they might not fix deep or severe issues. If you find that stress is affecting your physical health, relationships, or mental well-being, it is wise to reach out to a counselor or doctor. They can guide you toward additional treatments or strategies.

7.13 Final Thoughts on Stress and Essential Oils

Essential oils can be a gentle companion in handling stress. They are easy to use, they smell pleasant, and they can bring moments of relaxation into a busy day. By choosing the right oils and using them safely, you can add a small, helpful tool to your overall plan for a calmer life. Remember to pay attention to your own body and mind, and adjust as needed.

CHAPTER 8: Essential Oils for Sleep and Rest

8.1 The Importance of Good Sleep

Sleep is vital for a healthy life. During sleep, your body repairs cells, sorts through the day's events in your mind, and restores energy. Without enough rest, you might feel grouchy, have trouble remembering things, or even lower your body's ability to fight off sickness.

Many people struggle with falling or staying asleep. They might toss and turn or wake up feeling unrested. Essential oils can help create a setting that guides you toward better sleep. Used alongside good habits, they might improve the feeling of relaxation before bed.

8.2 Common Sleep Issues

1. **Trouble Falling Asleep**: You lie in bed, but your mind will not settle.
2. **Waking Up Often**: You fall asleep fine but wake up multiple times.
3. **Not Feeling Rested**: You sleep a normal number of hours but still feel tired.
4. **Shift Work Schedules**: Some jobs require you to sleep during the day, which can conflict with your body's natural rhythm.

Sometimes these problems are short-term, due to worry or a big change in your life. Other times, they might be long-term conditions like insomnia. If you suspect a serious issue, talk with a doctor. For mild sleep problems, certain essential oils can be part of a bedtime routine.

8.3 Brain Chemistry and Sleep

When you rest, your brain releases signals that tell the body to slow down. Melatonin is a hormone that helps regulate when you feel sleepy or awake. Stress hormones like cortisol can throw this off if they remain high at night. Scents that calm the mind may ease tension and guide the body into a restful state.

Some essential oils have molecules thought to calm the nervous system or support the parasympathetic state (the "rest and digest" mode). While the science is still growing, many people find these scents helpful.

8.4 Essential Oils Linked to Better Sleep

Several oils are popular for nighttime use:

1. **Lavender (Lavandula angustifolia)**
    - Possibly the most well-known for sleep support.
    - Mild floral scent that many people find soothing.
2. **Roman Chamomile (Chamaemelum nobile)**
    - Gentle, warm aroma.
    - Can be used for both stress and bedtime.
3. **Clary Sage (Salvia sclarea)**
    - Earthy, slightly sweet scent.
    - Some studies show it might have a comforting effect on the mind.
4. **Vetiver (Vetiveria zizanioides)**
    - Rich, earthy scent.
    - May calm racing thoughts, though it has a strong aroma that not everyone likes.
5. **Marjoram (Origanum majorana)**
    - Herb-like scent.
    - Linked to a soothing effect on the nervous system.
6. **Cedarwood (Cedrus atlantica or Juniperus virginiana)**
    - Woodsy, calming scent.
    - Often used to help ground the mind before bed.

You can use these alone or combine them in blends. Always consider your personal preferences. If you dislike a scent, it might have the opposite effect and keep you awake.

8.5 Safe Methods for Nighttime Use

1. **Bedside Diffuser**
    - Put a diffuser next to your bed.
    - Add 3–5 drops of an oil or blend.
    - Run it for about 15–30 minutes before turning off.

- Make sure it has an automatic shut-off feature if you keep it on while resting.
2. **Pillow Mist**
    - Mix 10-15 drops of a calming oil in 2 ounces of water or witch hazel.
    - Mist lightly on your pillow or sheets. Test on a small corner first to avoid stains.
3. **Aromatherapy Roll-On**
    - Blend 2-3 drops of your chosen sleep oil in a teaspoon of carrier oil.
    - Put it in a roll-on bottle.
    - Apply to wrists or the back of your neck about 30 minutes before bed.
4. **Bath**
    - Add 5-8 drops of an oil blend to a tablespoon of carrier oil or liquid soap.
    - Stir it into a warm bath.
    - Soak for at least 15 minutes to let your muscles relax.
5. **Inhalation**
    - If you do not want a room diffuser, you can put 1-2 drops of oil on a cotton ball near your pillow.
    - Do not put it too close to your face to avoid irritation.

8.6 Rare Tips for Improving Sleep Quality

- **Timing**: Using an oil right before bed is helpful, but also consider diffusing a gentle scent during your evening routine. This sends early signals to your brain that it is time to slow down.
- **Layering**: Combine a foot massage with a favorite calming oil and a warm pair of socks. The act of massaging feet can help quiet the mind.
- **Focusing on Breathing**: While you inhale a calming scent, practice slow breathing in bed. Count to four on the inhale, pause, then exhale for four. This can help clear thoughts.
- **Alternating Blends**: If you use the same oil every single night, you might grow used to it. Change scents or blends occasionally.
- **Mindful Lighting**: Dim the lights or use a soft lamp to set the mood for rest. Bright lights can keep your brain alert.

8.7 Supporting Habits for Better Rest

Essential oils alone may not be enough if you have poor sleep habits. Pair them with:

- **Regular Bedtime**: Sleeping and waking at the same time each day helps set your body clock.
- **No Electronics Before Bed**: Blue light from phones or tablets can disrupt melatonin. Try to stop using them at least 30 minutes before sleep.
- **Avoid Heavy Meals Late**: Eating a large meal close to bedtime can keep your body active.
- **Cut Down on Caffeine**: Coffee, tea, and soda can stay in your system for hours, making it harder to wind down.
- **Calming Activities**: Gentle reading, light stretching, or listening to soft music can prepare your mind for rest.

8.8 Sleep-Boosting Blends

1. **Classic Bedtime Blend**
    - Lavender: 3 drops
    - Cedarwood: 2 drops
    - Roman Chamomile: 2 drops
    - Diffuse for 20 minutes before turning in.
2. **Herbal Comfort Blend**
    - Clary Sage: 2 drops
    - Marjoram: 2 drops
    - Bergamot (furanocoumarin-free): 2 drops
    - Good for an evening foot massage with carrier oil.
3. **Earthy Deep Sleep Blend**
    - Vetiver: 1 drop
    - Lavender: 2 drops
    - Sweet Orange: 2 drops
    - Diffuse or use in a small personal inhaler. Vetiver can be strong, so if you do not like the aroma, reduce it to half a drop (dip a toothpick in the oil and swirl it in the blend).

8.9 Potential Pitfalls

- **Overstimulation**: Using too much oil or a scent that is too sharp (like strong mints or bright citrus) might keep you awake. Choose softer, more mellow aromas for nighttime.
- **Allergic Reactions**: Always patch test if you plan to apply the oil to your skin.
- **Messing Up Your Routine**: If you try a new blend every night, your body might get confused. Give a blend a few days to see if it helps.
- **Expecting Instant Results**: Essential oils can help you settle, but if you have chronic insomnia, you might need deeper treatment.
- **Inconsistent Habits**: If you only use oils but still stare at a bright screen late at night, the oils may not overcome that habit.

8.10 Helping Children and Older Adults

- **Children**
    - Choose mild oils like lavender or chamomile.
    - Use a low dilution (0.25% to 0.5%) if applying on skin, or diffuse a small amount in a spacious room.
    - Check with a doctor for very young children, especially under two years old.
- **Older Adults**
    - Skin can be thinner, so maintain a low dilution to prevent irritation.
    - Some older adults might be on medications, so check for possible interactions if ingesting or using large amounts.
    - Gentle diffusion is often enough to create a peaceful atmosphere.

8.11 Linking Sleep to Overall Well-Being

When you rest well, you have more energy, better focus, and likely a better mood. This can improve how you deal with daytime tasks. Essential oils can help set the stage for healthy sleep, but remember to address other factors like stress, exercise, and nutrition.

For instance, an evening walk, followed by a warm shower, then a short diffuser session with lavender, can create a smooth path to slumber. Experiment with small changes to see how your sleep improves.

8.12 Tips for Shift Workers

Shift workers often struggle to sleep during the day and stay awake at night. To help:

1. **Dark Room**: Use blackout curtains or an eye mask to mimic night during daylight hours.
2. **Noise Control**: Consider earplugs or a white noise machine.
3. **Strategic Use of Oils**: Diffuse grounding oils like cedarwood or vetiver before you lie down.
4. **Calming Routine**: Even though it is daytime, pretend it is your "night." Avoid bright screens right before bed.

This can trick the body into a rest mode despite daytime light.

8.13 Tracking Your Progress

It helps to keep a small sleep journal for a week or two:

- Note the oils you used and how you used them (diffuser, bath, etc.).
- Write down the time you went to bed and how long it took to fall asleep.
- Record any nighttime awakenings.
- Rate how rested you feel upon waking.

Looking at these notes can show if a certain oil or blend is making a difference. If you see an improvement, keep that method. If not, you might try a new combination or look at other factors (like cutting screen time or adjusting your bedtime).

8.14 Handling Occasional Restlessness

Even people who usually sleep well might have off nights. When this happens:

1. **Get Up Briefly**: If you cannot fall asleep after 20 minutes, sometimes it helps to get out of bed, walk around quietly, or read a few pages of a calming book.
2. **Deep Breathing**: Take slow, steady breaths to slow your heart rate.

3. **Light Aromatherapy**: Smell a calming oil from a cotton ball or roll-on, then try lying down again.

8.15 Rare Details About Sleep and Oils

- **Night Sweats**: Some women dealing with hormonal changes find clary sage or geranium supportive when experiencing night sweats. They might use a small diffuser by the bed.
- **Snoring Partners**: If snoring disrupts your rest, an oil like eucalyptus or thyme (properly diluted) may help clear breathing passages for the one who snores. This might reduce noise, though results vary.
- **Cool vs. Warm Blends**: Some oils have a "cooling" effect (like peppermint), while others feel "warming" (like ginger). For bedtime, it is usually best to avoid strong cooling oils unless they help you personally.

8.16 Combining with Other Relaxation Techniques

- **Guided Imagery**: Imagine a calm scene while inhaling a pleasant bedtime oil.
- **Gentle Yoga**: A few easy poses can stretch tight muscles. Diffuse a soft blend in the room.
- **Progressive Muscle Tension Release**: Tighten and relax muscle groups from toes to head, while breathing in a relaxing scent.

8.17 Staying Safe

- **Fire Hazards**: If using a candle diffuser, do not leave it burning while you sleep.
- **Skin Safety**: If you decide to apply an oil to your temples or behind your ears, always dilute.
- **Pet Safety**: If pets sleep in your room, pick oils that are not harmful to them and ensure good airflow.
- **Allergies**: Watch out for any signs of irritation.

8.18 When Sleep Issues Persist

If you follow good habits and try supportive oils but still cannot rest well, consult a professional. Long-lasting insomnia can have a range of causes, including stress disorders, hormonal changes, or hidden health issues. Essential oils can still be part of your plan, but you might also need medical advice or therapy.

8.19 Recommended Simple Blends to Experiment With

1. **Soft Dreams Roll-On**
    - 5 mL carrier oil (such as fractionated coconut oil)
    - 1 drop lavender
    - 1 drop marjoram
    - 1 drop roman chamomile
    - Roll on wrists or pulse points 30 minutes before bed.
2. **Deep Calm Inhaler**
    - Inhaler with cotton wick
    - 3 drops clary sage
    - 2 drops sweet orange
    - 1 drop cedarwood
    - Inhale gently for a few seconds before bed.
3. **Soothing Foot Rub**
    - 1 tablespoon unscented lotion or carrier oil
    - 2 drops lavender
    - 2 drops frankincense
    - Massage into feet before putting on soft socks.

8.20 Conclusion

Essential oils can be a helpful part of a bedtime routine, offering a gentle nudge toward rest. When used correctly, oils like lavender, chamomile, and cedarwood can help set a relaxing mood. Pair them with healthy habits like dim lighting, avoiding late-night screens, and keeping a consistent schedule. Over time, you might find you fall asleep faster or wake up less often.

Still, keep in mind that essential oils are not a solution for serious sleep conditions on their own. If your troubles continue, reach out to a healthcare professional. Used wisely, essential oils can help you wind down, calm the mind, and encourage more restful nights.

CHAPTER 9: Essential Oils for Mood and Emotional Support

9.1 Understanding Mood and Emotions

Mood and emotions play a large part in everyday life. Sometimes they feel light and positive. Other times they might be heavier and harder to manage. When people look for ways to support emotional well-being, they might try talking with friends, therapy, exercise, or meditation. Essential oils can also be part of that toolbox.

Our emotions can shift quickly based on triggers like events, memories, or even smells. A single scent might bring back a favorite memory, changing how you feel in that moment. Essential oils harness the power of smells by allowing you to breathe in natural fragrances that could help the mind and body feel calmer or brighter.

9.2 How Smell Affects Emotions

When you breathe in a scent, you inhale tiny odor molecules. These molecules interact with smell receptors in your nose, which send signals to the limbic system in the brain. The limbic system is linked to emotion, motivation, and memory. This is why certain smells can remind you of childhood or lift your spirits suddenly.

Not all scents have the same effect on everyone. A smell that helps one person feel happier might be too strong or unpleasant for someone else. That is why it is helpful to experiment with different essential oils to find which ones make you feel good and which ones do not.

9.3 Common Emotional States and Possible Oils

Essential oils can play a small but meaningful part in supporting different moods. Here are some common emotional states and popular oils people use to address them:

1. **Feeling Low or Sad**
   - **Citrus Oils (Orange, Grapefruit, Lemon)**: They often have bright, uplifting aromas.
   - **Geranium**: A floral scent that some say helps bring balance to the mind.
   - **Rose**: A rich floral scent sometimes linked to comfort.
2. **Feeling Stuck or Unmotivated**
   - **Peppermint**: Sharp and refreshing, can offer a quick mental spark.
   - **Rosemary**: Herbal and clear, often used for focus.
   - **Basil**: Another herb-like smell that might help the mind feel refreshed.
3. **Feeling Overwhelmed or Anxious**
   - **Lavender**: Known for calm support.
   - **Frankincense**: Deep, resinous scent that might help slow down racing thoughts.
   - **Bergamot (furanocoumarin-free if for skin)**: Light citrus smell that can ease tension for some.
4. **Feeling Irritated or Angry**
   - **Chamomile (Roman or German)**: Gentle, soothing aroma.
   - **Sandalwood**: Woody and smooth, sometimes used for grounding.
   - **Vetiver**: Earthy base note that can help settle intense emotions.
5. **Needing Encouragement or Comfort**
   - **Sweet Marjoram**: Warm herbal scent that some find comforting.
   - **Jasmine Absolute**: Floral, sweet, often used for emotional uplift.
   - **Clary Sage**: Earthy, somewhat floral, sometimes used for easing emotional tension.

9.4 Simple Ways to Use Essential Oils for Emotional Support

1. **Inhalation**
   - Place a drop or two of an oil on a tissue.
   - Hold it near your nose and breathe in slowly.
   - This quick method can be used when you feel an emotional shift coming.

2. **Diffusion**
   - Use a water-based diffuser or a fan diffuser in the room.
   - Add 3-5 drops of an oil or blend.
   - Let the aroma spread for 20-30 minutes.
   - Good for a living room or workspace.
3. **Personal Inhaler**
   - A small plastic or metal tube with a cotton wick inside.
   - Add 5-10 drops of essential oil to the wick.
   - Close it up and keep it in your bag or pocket.
   - Inhale gently when you need emotional support.
4. **Topical Application**
   - Dilute your chosen oil in a carrier oil (like sweet almond) at around 1-3%.
   - Apply to wrists, temples, or behind the ears.
   - Inhale the aroma that lingers on the skin.
5. **Room or Linen Sprays**
   - Mix 10-15 drops of essential oil with 1 ounce of water or witch hazel in a spray bottle.
   - Shake well and spray around the room or on pillows.
   - Helps set a calm or cheerful mood.

9.5 Rare Tips for Emotional Support

- **Morning Routine Boost**: Add a drop of a favorite citrus oil or peppermint to a corner of your shower floor. The steam can carry the scent, giving you an uplifting start to the day.
- **Emotional First Aid Kit**: Prepare small vials of different emotional support blends (like "Calm," "Focus," "Cheerful"). Label them. Use them when specific moods arise.
- **Pairing with Affirmations**: Some people find it helpful to speak or think positive statements while inhaling an oil. This connects a supportive thought with a comforting scent.
- **Timing**: If you know a stressful event is coming (like a job interview), try using an oil blend for calm about 15 minutes before, so the supportive effect can be in place by the time you start.
- **Environmental Scent Shifts**: If you work in an office, place a personal inhaler in your desk. Take small sniff breaks to prevent emotional buildup throughout the day.

9.6 Creating Blends for Mood Support

Blending oils can bring different scent notes together to shape an emotional effect. Here are a few ideas:

1. **Uplifting Blend**
    - Orange: 4 drops
    - Peppermint: 2 drops
    - Geranium: 1 drop
    - Use in a diffuser or personal inhaler to brighten the atmosphere.
2. **Balancing Blend**
    - Frankincense: 3 drops
    - Lavender: 3 drops
    - Clary Sage: 2 drops
    - Good for easing tension or feeling more at peace.
3. **Soothing Blend**
    - Chamomile (Roman): 2 drops
    - Sandalwood: 2 drops
    - Bergamot: 2 drops
    - Ideal for moments of irritability or frustration.

Adjust the number of drops based on how strong you want the scent to be. Also consider personal preference. Some might like more citrus notes, others more floral or woodsy notes.

9.7 Safety Points for Emotional Use

- **Avoid Over-Inhaling**: Even pleasant scents can feel overwhelming if used too often or in a small space with no ventilation.
- **Check for Allergies**: If you plan to apply oils on your skin, do a patch test first.
- **Be Mindful Around Others**: Some coworkers, family members, or friends might not enjoy certain scents. Let them know before diffusing in shared rooms.
- **Seek Professional Help**: Oils can help with mild emotional ups and downs, but if you have deeper concerns like depression, severe anxiety, or other issues, talk with a professional.

9.8 Incorporating Essential Oils into Daily Routines

Adding essential oils into daily habits can make them more effective:

1. **Morning Pep**
   - Use a bright, fresh scent in your shower or diffuser as you get ready.
   - This can help start the day in a positive way.
2. **Work Break Calm**
   - Carry a personal inhaler with a calming blend.
   - When you take a quick break, inhale slowly for a few breaths.
3. **Afternoon Pick-Me-Up**
   - Use a citrus or mint oil in a diffuser after lunch to keep energy levels steady without turning to too much caffeine.
4. **Evening Wind-Down**
   - Switch to deeper, more grounding oils like vetiver or sandalwood as night approaches.
   - Pair them with a relaxing activity like reading or a gentle hobby.

9.9 Emotional Well-Being for Children

Children also experience strong emotions. Essential oils should be used gently and with caution around them:

- **Choose Mild Oils**: Lavender or sweet orange at a low dilution (0.25–0.5%) can be enough.
- **Use a Diffuser in a Larger Room**: Avoid small, closed spaces.
- **Let Them Smell the Cap**: Have them smell the bottle's cap to see if they like it before diffusing.
- **Watch for Reactions**: If they get fussy, have watery eyes, or seem uncomfortable, turn off the diffuser and air out the room.

9.10 Supporting Older Adults

Older adults may have certain emotional needs, such as dealing with loneliness or adjusting to life changes. Some points to keep in mind:

- **Gentle Scents**: Strong smells might be too much for sensitive noses.
- **Check Medications**: Ensure no interactions if they apply oils on the skin, though this risk is usually small.
- **Diffuse in Common Areas**: A living room diffuser with a light floral or citrus blend can enhance a sense of calm.
- **Personal Scent Items**: A lightly scented pillow or small inhaler can help if someone feels anxious or restless at night.

9.11 Combining Essential Oils with Other Emotional Tools

- **Music Therapy**: Light background music plus a calming essential oil in a diffuser can double the soothing effect.
- **Physical Activities**: Yoga or gentle stretching with a mild, grounding scent can help the mind relax.
- **Creative Work**: Painting, writing, or coloring while breathing in a pleasant aroma may help unlock more creativity and reduce stress.
- **Counseling Sessions**: Some counselors or therapists use essential oils in waiting rooms or during sessions to help clients settle.

9.12 Handling Emotional Ups and Downs Over Time

Emotional well-being is not a straight line. You might feel great one week, and then life events throw you off the next. Essential oils can be a steady friend, giving you small moments of relief. But remember, they do not replace professional help if you have intense or lasting emotional challenges.

9.13 Helpful Habits Alongside Essential Oils

1. **Stay Hydrated**: Thirst can make you feel tired or less clear-headed.
2. **Eat Balanced Meals**: Nutritional imbalances might worsen mood swings.
3. **Get Regular Movement**: A walk or simple exercise can increase endorphins.
4. **Limit Caffeine and Sugar**: These can create spikes and crashes in mood.

5. **Practice Gratitude**: Writing down a few good things each day may shift the mind toward a positive outlook.

9.14 Addressing Group Dynamics

If you plan to diffuse oils in a setting with multiple people, like a family gathering or office:

- **Ask if Anyone Objects**: Someone might have an allergy or asthma.
- **Pick Gentle, Universal Favorites**: Oils like sweet orange, lemon, or lavender are often more acceptable to groups than strong ones like patchouli or ylang ylang.
- **Diffuse for Short Periods**: 15-20 minutes every couple of hours can be enough to refresh the space without overpowering it.

9.15 When Emotions Get Overwhelming

If you find essential oils do not help enough, or if your feelings of sadness, worry, or anger become extreme:

- **Talk to a Professional**: A counselor, therapist, or doctor can give guidance.
- **Check on Physical Health**: Sometimes thyroid issues, vitamin deficiencies, or hormonal imbalances can affect mood.
- **Reach Out to Friends or Family**: Sharing struggles with people you trust can be part of healing.

9.16 Creating a Personal Mood Journal

To learn which oils work best for you, consider making a mood journal:

1. **Daily Note**: Write how you feel each morning and evening.
2. **Oil Used**: Include which oil or blend you inhaled or diffused.
3. **Method**: Note if it was a diffuser, inhaler, or topical use.
4. **Effect**: Did you feel calmer, brighter, or more focused afterward?
5. **Trends**: After a few weeks, look for patterns. Which oils helped the most?

A journal can help you build a personalized emotional toolkit.

9.17 Trying New Oils Cautiously

When branching out from familiar oils:

- **Purchase Small Sizes**: A 5 mL bottle is enough to see if you enjoy the scent.
- **Sniff from the Cap**: Get a sense of the aroma before deciding on further steps.
- **Blend with Known Favorites**: If an unfamiliar oil smells too strong alone, mix one drop with a few drops of a favorite oil to balance it out.
- **Observe Effects**: Notice if it makes you feel relaxed, energetic, or neutral.

9.18 Rare Facts about Emotional Support Oils

- **Jasmine at Night**: Some find that the scent of jasmine in the evening can be both comforting and slightly stimulating. It might help certain people feel balanced rather than drowsy.
- **Rose Geranium**: Different from standard geranium, rose geranium has a sweeter floral note, often used in mood-lifting blends.
- **Citrus Leaf Oils (Petitgrain)**: Oils from leaves of citrus trees (like petitgrain) carry a fresh, slightly floral smell that can be calming without being too sweet.

9.19 Sample Daily Emotional Support Schedule

- **Morning**: Diffuse a bright blend with sweet orange and peppermint for about 15 minutes.
- **Midday**: Use a personal inhaler with rosemary and lemon if you start feeling sluggish.
- **Late Afternoon**: If stress builds up, inhale a calming oil like lavender or chamomile.
- **Evening**: Diffuse a grounding blend of sandalwood and bergamot for 20 minutes while reading or resting.
- **Night**: Use a gentle pillow spray with lavender to settle into sleep.

9.20 Conclusion

Essential oils can support a healthy emotional state by giving subtle but helpful shifts in how you feel. From uplifting citrus scents to grounding woodsy aromas, there are many ways to match oils to your mood needs. Keep in mind that people respond differently to scents, so take time to see which oils work best for you. Use them in combination with other good habits—like balanced nutrition, exercise, and, if needed, professional mental health advice.

By thoughtfully selecting and applying essential oils, you can create small moments of relief or joy in your day. Over time, these small moments can add up to a more stable mood. Remember that while essential oils are a nice addition, they are not a complete fix for deep emotional concerns. With wise choices and safe use, they can be a gentle ally in caring for your emotional wellness.

CHAPTER 10: Essential Oils for Skin and Beauty

10.1 Why Skin Care Matters

The skin is the body's largest organ. It protects you from the outside world, helps regulate temperature, and can reflect your overall health. Many people want smooth, healthy-looking skin, and this desire leads them to try different lotions, creams, or skincare routines.

Essential oils can be part of a skincare plan when used wisely. They provide natural scents and may offer benefits for certain skin types. But they are also powerful and might cause irritation if not handled with care. This chapter will explore ways to include essential oils in a beauty regimen without risking dryness or breakouts.

10.2 Basic Skin Types

People often classify skin into a few general categories, though real skin can be more complicated:

1. **Oily Skin**: Produces excess sebum, leading to a shiny look and possible clogged pores.
2. **Dry Skin**: Lacks enough moisture, can feel tight or appear flaky.
3. **Combination Skin**: Has oily areas (often the T-zone: forehead, nose, chin) and dry or normal areas elsewhere.
4. **Sensitive Skin**: Reacts easily to products, might turn red or feel itchy.
5. **Normal Skin**: Balanced sebum production, fewer breakouts, not too dry.

Knowing your general skin type can guide which oils or products might suit you better.

10.3 Common Essential Oils for Skin Care

1. **Tea Tree (Melaleuca alternifolia)**

- Known for its cleansing properties.
- Popular for oily or blemish-prone skin.
- Must be diluted before applying.

2. **Lavender (Lavandula angustifolia)**
   - Gentle, soothing oil.
   - May help with redness and minor irritations.
   - Works for many skin types, if diluted.
3. **Geranium (Pelargonium graveolens)**
   - Floral scent, often used for balancing skin's oil production.
   - May be suitable for both dry and oily areas.
4. **Chamomile (Roman or German)**
   - Gentle oil known for calming properties.
   - Good choice for sensitive or easily irritated skin.
5. **Frankincense (Boswellia carterii)**
   - Woody, resinous aroma.
   - Sometimes used for mature or dry skin.
   - Believed by some to help reduce the look of small lines.
6. **Rose (Rosa damascena)**
   - Luxurious floral aroma, can be pricey.
   - Often seen in high-end skincare for dry or mature skin.
   - A little goes a long way.
7. **Ylang Ylang (Cananga odorata)**
   - Sweet, heavy floral scent.
   - Sometimes used to balance oil production.
   - Use sparingly to avoid overpowering scent.
8. **Patchouli (Pogostemon cablin)**
   - Earthy aroma.
   - Some people use it for dry, chapped skin.
   - Strong smell, so only a small amount is needed.

10.4 Carrier Oils for Skin Application

To use essential oils on the skin, dilute them in a carrier oil. Some common carriers include:

1. **Jojoba Oil**
   - Similar to the skin's natural sebum.
   - Good for most skin types, may help balance oily areas.
2. **Sweet Almond Oil**

- Light texture, commonly used.
- Good for normal to dry skin.
3. **Argan Oil**
    - Rich in vitamin E.
    - Often used for mature or dry skin, but can be heavy for some.
4. **Rosehip Oil**
    - Contains essential fatty acids.
    - Favored for scar-prone or mature skin.
5. **Fractionated Coconut Oil**
    - Clear, odorless, light.
    - Common in homemade skincare blends.

Pick a carrier oil based on your skin needs. For oily skin, a lighter carrier like jojoba might be better. For very dry skin, something richer like argan might help.

10.5 Dilution Guidelines for Skin Care

A safe general range for facial products is about 0.5% to 1% essential oil in the final mixture. This means:

- **0.5%** = 1 drop of essential oil per 2 teaspoons (10 mL) of carrier oil.
- **1%** = 1 drop of essential oil per 1 teaspoon (5 mL) of carrier oil.

For body oils or lotions, you can go up to about 2–3%, but if you have sensitive skin or a known reaction, stay on the lower side. Always patch test a new blend on a small area of skin (like the inside of your wrist) and wait 24 hours to check for irritation.

10.6 Building a Simple Skincare Routine with Essential Oils

1. **Cleanse**
    - Start with a gentle facial cleanser suitable for your skin type.
    - Avoid harsh scrubbing, which can irritate skin.
2. **Tone**
    - Use a toner that helps balance the skin's pH.
    - Some people like hydrosols (flower waters) such as rose or lavender hydrosol.

3. **Moisturize**
   - Mix a drop of your chosen essential oil in a small amount of carrier oil or unscented lotion.
   - Gently massage onto skin.
4. **Spot Treatments**
   - For blemishes, a drop of tea tree diluted in carrier oil dabbed on the spot might help.
   - For dry patches, add a bit of frankincense or chamomile in a heavier carrier oil.
5. **Weekly Mask or Scrub**
   - You can create a simple scrub with sugar or ground oats plus a bit of carrier oil and a drop of essential oil.
   - Or apply a clay mask to absorb excess oils, adding 1–2 drops of skin-friendly essential oil.

10.7 Specific Skin Concerns

1. **Blemish-Prone Skin**
   - Tea tree, lavender, and geranium can be helpful.
   - Avoid overwashing, which can strip skin and cause more oil production.
2. **Dry, Flaky Areas**
   - Frankincense, rose, and patchouli might support the skin's moisture barrier.
   - Use richer carrier oils, and consider a thicker balm at night.
3. **Sensitive or Redness-Prone Skin**
   - Chamomile, lavender, and rose are gentle choices.
   - Patch test carefully, and stick to very low dilutions.
4. **Mature Skin**
   - Frankincense, rose, and ylang ylang are often included in products aimed at smoothing the look of fine lines.
   - A serum with argan or rosehip oil can be applied before bed.
5. **Dull Skin**
   - Geranium or a mild citrus oil (like sweet orange) at a low dilution might help brighten.
   - Consider limiting sun exposure when using citrus oils due to possible phototoxicity (unless it's a furanocoumarin-free version).

10.8 Rare Tips for Skin Care with Essential Oils

- **Chill Your Tools**: Storing a jade roller or gua sha tool in the fridge can add a cool effect when massaging essential oil blends onto the face.
- **Night vs. Day Use**: Some oils (like citrus) are best used at night if they cause photosensitivity.
- **Steam Facial**: Add 1–2 drops of an oil like chamomile or lavender to a bowl of hot water. Lean over (not too close), drape a towel over your head, and let the steam open your pores for about 5 minutes.
- **Use Glass Containers**: Store your DIY blends in dark glass bottles to protect them from light and oxidation.
- **Keep It Simple**: Too many products can overwhelm the skin. Pick a few steps that work and stay consistent.

10.9 Body and Hair Care

Essential oils are not just for the face. They can be used for body or hair routines, too.

1. **Body Oils**
   - Make a body oil blend by mixing 4–6 drops of an oil like lavender or geranium per tablespoon (15 mL) of carrier oil.
   - Apply after a bath or shower to help lock in moisture.
2. **Bath Soaks**
   - Mix 5–8 drops of essential oil with a tablespoon of carrier oil or liquid soap before adding to the bath.
   - Soak for about 15 minutes.
3. **Hair Masks**
   - Add 2–3 drops of rosemary oil to a tablespoon of coconut or argan oil.
   - Massage into your scalp and hair, leave for 20 minutes, then shampoo.
   - Some believe rosemary may help with hair appearance.
4. **Foot Care**
   - Tea tree or peppermint diluted in a carrier oil can freshen feet.
   - A foot soak with Epsom salts plus a drop of lavender can relax tired feet.

10.10 DIY Beauty Recipes

1. **Facial Serum for Dry Skin**
   - 1 tablespoon argan oil
   - 1 tablespoon jojoba oil
   - 2 drops frankincense
   - 1 drop rose (optional)
   - Store in a 1 oz dropper bottle, use 2–3 drops on face at night.
2. **Balancing Facial Toner**
   - 2 ounces witch hazel (alcohol-free if possible)
   - 2 ounces distilled water
   - 3 drops geranium
   - 2 drops lavender
   - Shake before use, apply with a cotton pad to clean skin.
3. **Soothing Body Butter**
   - 1/2 cup shea butter
   - 2 tablespoons sweet almond oil
   - Gently melt and stir, let it cool slightly
   - Add 5 drops lavender and 3 drops chamomile
   - Whip with a handheld mixer until fluffy, store in a jar.
4. **Calming Lip Balm**
   - 1 tablespoon beeswax pellets
   - 1 tablespoon coconut oil
   - 1 tablespoon shea butter
   - Melt slowly over low heat
   - Add 2 drops of peppermint or lavender before pouring into lip balm containers.

10.11 Avoiding Irritation and Breakouts

Even gentle oils can cause problems if used in high amounts or if your skin is sensitive. Follow these guidelines:

- **Patch Test**: Always apply a small amount of the product on your wrist or behind your ear. Wait 24 hours.
- **Mind Heavy Oils**: Some carriers (like coconut oil) might clog pores for some people. Test them slowly.

- **Watch Out for Expiry**: Old oils can oxidize and may irritate the skin.
- **Do Not Overuse Essential Oils**: More drops do not mean better results. Stick to recommended dilutions.

10.12 Handling Acne or Breakouts

For those with acne:

- **Spot Treatment**: Dilute tea tree or lavender in a carrier oil. Use a cotton swab to dab on blemishes.
- **Gentle Products**: Avoid harsh scrubs that can tear the skin.
- **Do Not Pick**: Picking leads to scarring. Let the blemish heal with supportive skincare.
- **Lifestyle Factors**: Acne can also be linked to diet, hormones, or stress. Consider a balanced approach.

10.13 Supporting Mature Skin

As skin ages, it may become thinner, drier, and lose elasticity:

- **Nourishing Serums**: Add oils like rose, frankincense, or ylang ylang in a rich carrier oil.
- **Gentle Cleansers**: Use mild, non-stripping products.
- **Hydration**: Drink enough water and eat foods with healthy fats.
- **Sun Protection**: A sunscreen is key, as sun damage can speed up signs of aging.

10.14 Addressing Dark Spots or Uneven Tone

Some individuals want to reduce the appearance of dark spots or even out skin tone. Oils like frankincense, geranium, or a small amount of carrot seed oil might be used in a carrier. However, results vary, and it might take weeks or months to see any change. Also, be cautious with photosensitive oils, as they might worsen dark spots if you go in the sun without protection.

10.15 Hair and Scalp Tips

1. **Scalp Massage**
   - Mix 3 drops rosemary and 2 drops lavender in 1 tablespoon of jojoba oil.
   - Gently massage into the scalp.
   - Leave for a bit before rinsing.
2. **Avoid Overwashing**
   - Washing hair too often can strip natural oils.
   - A mild shampoo without harsh chemicals is kinder to both hair and scalp.
3. **Split Ends**
   - Condition the tips with a bit of argan oil plus 1 drop of ylang ylang.
   - Trim split ends regularly to maintain a neater look.

10.16 Rare Facts for Beauty Care

- **Green Clay Masks**: Adding 1 drop of essential oil like lavender to a green clay mask can offer a clarifying treatment for oily or combination skin.
- **Honey Face Wash**: A gentle honey face wash (using raw honey) plus 1 drop of tea tree or lavender can be a mild cleansing option.
- **Sun-Damaged Skin**: Some people turn to lavender and chamomile in a cool compress for mild relief, though sunburn is best prevented with sunscreen and protective clothing.
- **Storing DIY Products**: Keep them in the fridge if they contain fresh ingredients (like aloe gel), but be aware the mix might thicken in cold temperature.

10.17 Using Essential Oils in Makeup

While many commercial makeup products have synthetic fragrances, you can find or create your own items with essential oils:

- **Lip Gloss**: A drop of peppermint or orange oil in a base of castor oil and beeswax can add subtle scent.

- **Setting Spray**: A small spray bottle with distilled water, witch hazel, and 1–2 drops of lavender or geranium can lightly refresh makeup.
- **Avoid Eye Area**: Do not put essential oils too close to the eyes, as they can cause irritation.

10.18 Eco-Friendly and Ethical Concerns

If you care about the source of your products:

- **Organic Oils and Carriers**: These may reduce exposure to pesticides.
- **Fair Trade**: Some carrier oils like shea butter or argan oil might be available as fair trade, helping communities where they are produced.
- **Sustainability**: Certain essential oils come from plants at risk of overharvesting. Ensure the brand you buy from practices responsible sourcing.

10.19 Troubleshooting Skin Problems

- **Unexpected Breakouts**: If you get pimples after trying a new oil blend, stop using it and let the skin calm down.
- **Redness or Rash**: Wash the area with mild soap and water. If it persists, contact a healthcare provider.
- **Dry or Tight Feeling**: Increase carrier oil or switch to a richer one. You might also lower the essential oil drops if they are causing sensitivity.
- **Greasy Look**: Try a lighter carrier or reduce the amount of oil you apply. You can blot excess oil with a tissue.

10.20 Conclusion

Using essential oils in your skincare and beauty routine can add pleasant scents and potential benefits. Oils like tea tree, lavender, geranium, and frankincense have a long history in skin care. But always remember that essential oils are powerful, and improper use can harm the skin. Follow safe dilution guidelines, choose oils suited to your skin type, and patch test any new product.

At the same time, take care of the basics: gentle cleansing, balanced hydration, sun protection, and a good diet. Essential oils can act as an extra step that boosts your routine, but they are not a replacement for overall skin health practices. With mindful choices and some experimentation, you can enjoy the sweet or herbal aromas while giving your skin a natural touch. If problems persist or you have major concerns, consult a dermatologist or another qualified professional.

Essential oils for skin and beauty can be a fun and rewarding path, letting you craft products that suit your personal style and skin needs. Keep things simple, be consistent in usage, and pay attention to how your skin responds. Over time, you might discover wonderful blends that become treasured parts of your daily self-care.

CHAPTER 11: Essential Oils for Children and the Elderly

11.1 Special Care for Different Ages

Children and older adults often have different bodies and needs. Their skin can be thinner, and their sense of smell might be more sensitive or less sharp. Some might have breathing concerns or be on medications. Because of these differences, it is good to know safe ways to use essential oils with children and older adults.

In this chapter, we will look at which oils might be helpful for little ones and seniors. We will also talk about safety rules, how to dilute oils, and when to get medical advice.

11.2 Why Children Need Careful Handling of Essential Oils

Children's bodies and skin are still growing. Their liver and kidneys might not break down certain substances as well as an adult's can. Also, they often weigh less than adults, so a small amount of essential oil can have a bigger effect on them. Here are some common issues to keep in mind:

1. **Sensitive Skin**: Children's skin can react more quickly to strong products.
2. **Stronger Reaction to Smells**: Kids might find a scent too strong even if an adult feels it is mild.
3. **Possibility of Accidental Swallowing**: Curious kids might put things in their mouth, so storing oils out of reach is vital.

Taking these concerns into account can help you use essential oils in a safer way. Never forget that "natural" does not automatically mean "safe in any amount." Always follow correct methods and keep an eye on how the child reacts.

11.3 General Safety Guidelines for Children

1. **Age Restrictions**: Many experts recommend limiting the use of essential oils for babies under three months old. For older infants and toddlers, only mild oils and very low dilutions are advised. Always check with a pediatrician if you have doubts.
2. **Dilution Rates**: While adults often use a 1–3% dilution for the skin, children usually need 0.25–1% at most. For very young kids (under two years), a 0.25% dilution can be enough.
3. **Patch Test**: Before applying any new blend to a child's skin, do a small test on the forearm or leg. Wait 24 hours to see if there is redness or itching.
4. **No Ingestion**: Avoid giving essential oils by mouth unless a qualified healthcare professional says it is safe (which is rare).
5. **Safe Storage**: Keep oils locked away or in a high cupboard. Children might be tempted to open and smell them, which can lead to spills or worse.
6. **Diffusion Rules**: If diffusing oils around children, start with a very small amount, and limit the time to about 15 minutes. Keep a door or window slightly open for air flow. Watch the child's behavior. If they seem bothered, stop immediately.

11.4 Essential Oils Commonly Used for Children

Here are some oils that many people consider gentler for kids, but always dilute them properly:

1. **Lavender (Lavandula angustifolia)**
    - Soft floral scent.
    - Often linked to a calm atmosphere.
    - Can be used in a bedtime routine (mild diffuser use or lightly diluted in a foot rub).
2. **Roman Chamomile (Chamaemelum nobile)**
    - Sweet, apple-like smell.
    - Known for its soothing qualities.
    - Suitable for mild skin care when diluted and for gentle bedtime help.

3. **Sweet Orange (Citrus sinensis)**
     - Bright, cheerful aroma.
     - Children often like this fruity smell.
     - Can be used in a diffuser during the day to help lift the mood.
4. **Mandarin (Citrus reticulata)**
     - Similar to sweet orange but with a slightly softer scent.
     - Good for a calm but pleasant environment.
     - Use carefully on skin due to possible light sensitivity if it is not a furanocoumarin-free type.
5. **Tea Tree (Melaleuca alternifolia)**
     - Stronger scent, so use less around children.
     - Sometimes used for small skin issues when properly diluted.
     - Keep an eye on the reaction because tea tree can be intense if overused.

Not all children like the same smells. If your child dislikes lavender, for example, do not force it. There are other gentle options.

11.5 Common Uses for Essential Oils in Childhood

1. **Calming Before Bed**: A few drops of lavender in a diffuser or a gentle foot massage with a chamomile blend can create a relaxing pre-sleep routine.
2. **Mild Skin Support**: If a child has minor skin irritation, a light application of chamomile or lavender (well-diluted) might help.
3. **Uplifting Mood**: Sweet orange in a diffuser can bring a friendly scent into a playroom.
4. **Minor Bumps**: Some parents use a cold compress with one drop of lavender or chamomile to soothe small scrapes or bruises, but always check for any sting or reaction.

Remember, these are gentle uses. For larger health problems or persistent symptoms, see a doctor.

11.6 Baby-Safe Approaches

Babies under three months generally should not have essential oils applied to their skin unless a medical professional approves it. Here are some safer ideas for the youngest ones:

1. **Gentle Diffusion**: If at all, use just 1–2 drops in a large, well-ventilated room for a short time. Observe the baby's response.
2. **Aromatic Clothing**: Put a drop of a gentle oil like lavender on a piece of cloth near (not on) the baby's crib, out of their reach, so they get a faint scent without direct contact.
3. **Mom or Dad's Clothing**: Some parents place a drop of a mild oil on their own shirt so the baby might smell it while being held, without the oil touching the baby's skin.

Always err on the side of caution. Babies are very sensitive, and it is better to use less or none if you are not sure.

11.7 Essential Oils to Use with Caution for Kids

Certain oils can be risky for children due to their potency or certain compounds:

- **Eucalyptus (especially Eucalyptus globulus)**: Strong. Some experts worry it can irritate a child's airways. If you use it, choose a species like Eucalyptus radiata at a very low dilution around older children, and avoid it for babies.
- **Peppermint (Mentha x piperita)**: Its high menthol content can cause breathing issues in infants or toddlers. Many recommend avoiding it for kids under six years old.
- **Cinnamon Bark (Cinnamomum verum)**: Hot and likely to irritate skin.
- **Clove (Syzygium aromaticum)**: Also hot and can be harsh on skin.

If in doubt, stick with gentler options like lavender or chamomile.

11.8 Extra Tips for Children

- **Make It Fun**: Let them pick between two mild scents if appropriate.
- **Avoid Overuse**: Using oils daily for long stretches might cause sensitivity. Give breaks.
- **Teach Safety**: Older kids can learn that essential oils are not to be played with or tasted.
- **Be Prepared**: In case of accidental ingestion or contact with eyes, rinse and contact a medical professional right away.

11.9 Essential Oils for the Elderly

Older adults may benefit from essential oils for issues like stiffness, occasional pain, or restlessness at night. Many older folks also enjoy pleasant scents that remind them of good memories. However, as people age, their skin can become more fragile, and they might have health conditions that require medication. We should be mindful of these factors:

- **Skin Fragility**: Lower dilution (about 0.5–1%) can reduce the chance of irritation.
- **Possible Breathing Concerns**: If someone has asthma or COPD, do not use strong diffusions that could trigger breathing issues.
- **Medication Interactions**: While topical use rarely affects prescription drugs, ingestion or very high usage might interfere with some medications, so caution is advised.

11.10 Common Oils for Older Adults

1. **Lavender (Lavandula angustifolia)**
   - Often used for easing tension and improving sleep quality.
   - Gentle and generally well-tolerated.
2. **Frankincense (Boswellia carterii)**
   - Woody scent that some find comforting.
   - Sometimes applied (diluted) to support the skin or used in a diffuser for calm.

3. **Roman Chamomile (Chamaemelum nobile)**
    - Helpful for individuals with sensitive skin or those who need a mild mood-lifting effect.
    - Can soothe minor irritations or restlessness.
4. **Sweet Marjoram (Origanum majorana)**
    - Herbal aroma that some older adults appreciate for muscle or joint comfort when diluted in a massage oil.
5. **Rose (Rosa damascena)**
    - Luxurious scent but can be expensive.
    - May bring a sense of comfort or emotional ease.

Again, each person's preferences will differ. Some older adults might not like strong smells, so keep it mild.

11.11 Ways Older Adults Might Use Essential Oils

1. **Gentle Diffusion**
    - Use 2-3 drops in a diffuser for 15-20 minutes at a time.
    - Helps refresh the air without becoming overpowering.
2. **Topical Massage**
    - Mix 1-2 drops of an oil in a tablespoon of carrier oil (like sweet almond or fractionated coconut).
    - Apply gently to hands, feet, or shoulders for relaxing support.
    - Good for older adults who experience dryness or want a mild soothing effect.
3. **Warm Compress**
    - Fill a bowl with warm water, add 1 drop of essential oil, soak a cloth, and apply it to stiff areas.
    - Always check water temperature to avoid burns.
4. **Aromatic Bath**
    - For those who can safely bathe without assistance, add 2-3 drops of an essential oil mixed in a tablespoon of carrier oil to the bath.
    - Make sure the bath is not too hot and that there is help if mobility is limited.

11.12 Concerns for Older Adults with Health Conditions

- **High Blood Pressure**: Some say to be careful with rosemary or thyme if a person has uncontrolled high blood pressure. While the evidence is not fully confirmed, it is wise to be cautious.
- **Blood Thinners**: Oils high in eugenol (like clove) might add to blood thinning effects.
- **Memory Changes**: People with dementia may become confused by strong smells. Keep it gentle and try known favorite scents instead of new ones that might be unfamiliar.

If an older person is on multiple medications, discuss any new essential oil routine with a pharmacist or doctor to rule out problems.

11.13 Emotional Well-Being for Seniors

Loneliness or stress can appear in older age. Pleasant scents can help lift mood or bring a sense of comfort. Some older adults may enjoy diffusing a comforting oil while looking through photo albums or during quiet time. Others might benefit from a simple hand massage with a mild scented oil to reduce stress and feel more relaxed.

Soft scents like lavender, chamomile, or sweet orange can be enough to brighten a mood. Sometimes the ritual of smelling a calming oil before bedtime can also help with restless nights.

11.14 Practical Tips for Caregivers

- **Communication**: If you care for a senior, ask about their scent preferences and watch for signs of discomfort.
- **Keep it Simple**: A single oil or a simple blend is often enough. Complex mixes might be confusing or too strong.

- **Avoid Slips**: If using oils in a bath or foot soak, clean the tub afterward. Oil residues can make surfaces slippery.
- **Store Safely**: Even seniors can accidentally ingest oils if their eyesight is poor and they mistake the bottle for something else. Label clearly and keep them out of regular food or drink areas.
- **Involve Them**: Let the older adult pick which oil they like, if they can. This can add a sense of control and enjoyment.

11.15 Rare Tips for Children and Older Adults Together

Sometimes children spend time with grandparents or older relatives. If you want to use essential oils in a shared environment:

- **Gentle Scents**: Choose oils that are mild for both age groups, like lavender or mandarin.
- **Minimal Diffusion**: Limit how long you diffuse to avoid overpowering anyone's senses.
- **No Confusion with Bottles**: Keep kids from picking them up, and ensure older adults with poor eyesight do not confuse the oil for something else.
- **Check Everyone's Reaction**: If anyone—child or senior—coughs, complains of headache, or shows discomfort, stop diffusing and air out the room.

11.16 Helpful Blends for Children

1. **Soothing Bedtime Blend**
    - 2 drops lavender
    - 1 drop Roman chamomile
    - Diffuse in a large room for 10–15 minutes before bed.
    - For a lotion blend, add 1 drop total of this mix to a teaspoon of carrier lotion for a preschooler (over two years old).
2. **Cheerful Playtime Blend**
    - 2 drops sweet orange
    - 1 drop mandarin

- 1 drop lavender (optional if you want a soft floral note)
- Use in a personal inhaler or diffuser in a large play area for a short time.
3. **Mild Skin Support Blend** (for small scrapes, over age two)
    - 1 drop tea tree
    - 1 drop lavender
    - Mix in 2 teaspoons of carrier oil.
    - Dab lightly on the area with clean hands.

11.17 Helpful Blends for Older Adults

1. **Joint Comfort Massage Oil**
    - 2 tablespoons carrier oil (like sweet almond)
    - 2 drops sweet marjoram
    - 2 drops lavender
    - Warm slightly in your hands and apply gently to stiff areas.
2. **Calming Evening Blend**
    - 2 drops frankincense
    - 2 drops lavender
    - Diffuse for 15 minutes before bedtime.
3. **Soothing Foot Soak**
    - A basin of warm water
    - 1 tablespoon Epsom salt
    - 2 drops Roman chamomile
    - 2 drops lavender (optional)
    - Stir and soak feet for 10–15 minutes, with help nearby if mobility is an issue.

11.18 Signs of Trouble

Whether for kids or older adults, watch out for:

- **Redness or Rash on Skin**: Could be an allergic reaction. Stop use and wash the area.

- **Breathing Problems**: If someone starts coughing, wheezing, or feels tightness in the chest, stop diffusion and move to fresh air.
- **Headaches or Dizziness**: Too-strong scents can cause discomfort. Ventilate the room immediately.
- **Confusion or Changes in Behavior**: If older adults act oddly after an oil is diffused, turn off the diffuser and assess the situation.

Seek professional advice if problems last or seem serious.

11.19 Joining Essential Oils with Other Support Methods

Essential oils are not the only path to comfort. Think of them as a piece of a bigger plan:

- **Kids**: Combine mild oils with plenty of rest, good nutrition, and a calm home environment.
- **Older Adults**: Pair light scented use with gentle exercise, social interaction, and medication management as directed by a doctor.

When used wisely with other tools—like reading bedtime stories for children or providing warm blankets for seniors—essential oils can add a pleasant touch to daily life.

11.20 Conclusion

Children and older adults can enjoy essential oils when handled with special care. The goal is to use gentle scents, lower dilution, and short diffusion times. If done correctly, essential oils can calm a restless child before bed or bring comfort to a grandparent's day. However, always be ready to stop if you see any negative reaction. Keep medical advice close at hand, especially if a person has health concerns or is very young.

By matching the right oil to the age, need, and personal taste, you can safely share the benefits of these natural aromas. Always remember that safety and moderation come first. When chosen and used properly, essential oils can bring a simple, comforting presence to daily routines for both children and older adults alike.

CHAPTER 12: Essential Oils in Household Cleaning

12.1 Introduction to Natural Cleaning

Many people want to reduce the amount of harsh chemicals in their homes. They might look for ways to keep surfaces clean and fresh without relying on strong artificial fragrances. Essential oils can help by adding fresh scents and some cleaning power. While they are not magic, they can complement simple ingredients like vinegar, baking soda, or soap to create pleasant cleaning solutions.

This chapter will explore ways to incorporate essential oils into daily chores. We will talk about safety, popular oils for cleaning, and how to make simple blends for kitchens, bathrooms, and more.

12.2 Why Use Essential Oils for Cleaning?

1. **Natural Aroma**: Many store-bought cleaners have strong artificial smells. Essential oils offer a plant-based scent.
2. **Extra Benefits**: Some oils have properties that can help limit certain types of unwanted microbes on surfaces.
3. **Personal Preference**: You can adjust the fragrance by choosing oils you enjoy.
4. **Reducing Chemical Load**: If you aim to keep your home environment simpler, essential oils combined with basic items like vinegar and baking soda can be a step in that direction.

However, remember that essential oils are still potent. While they are natural, they need proper handling to avoid harm.

12.3 Basic Cleaning Ingredients to Combine with Essential Oils

- **White Vinegar**: Often used to dissolve mineral deposits or remove grease. It has its own smell, but you can mask some of that with essential oils.
- **Baking Soda (Sodium Bicarbonate)**: Useful for scrubbing sinks or bathtubs. It can also help absorb odors in the fridge.
- **Liquid Castile Soap**: A gentle but effective soap that can clean floors, counters, and more.
- **Rubbing Alcohol (Isopropyl Alcohol)**: Sometimes used in homemade sprays to dry quickly and aid in sanitizing.
- **Water**: Distilled or boiled water can be a base for many DIY cleaners.

When you add essential oils to these items, you create an aromatic and basic cleaning solution. Still, know that homemade cleaners might not kill all pathogens as thoroughly as commercial disinfectants, so use them wisely.

12.4 Popular Essential Oils for Cleaning

1. **Lemon (Citrus limon)**
   - Bright, fresh scent that many people link with cleanliness.
   - Good in kitchen sprays or floor cleansers.
2. **Tea Tree (Melaleuca alternifolia)**
   - Sharp aroma, often used for its cleansing properties.
   - Great in bathroom cleaners or musty areas. Use in small amounts to avoid an overpowering smell.
3. **Peppermint (Mentha x piperita)**
   - Cool, minty aroma.
   - Can help freshen the air and repel some small insects.
   - May be too strong for some; test carefully.
4. **Eucalyptus (Eucalyptus radiata or Eucalyptus globulus)**
   - Clean, airy aroma.
   - Used in laundry or for cleaning floors.

- Ensure good ventilation, especially if someone in the home has breathing concerns.
5. **Lavender (Lavandula angustifolia)**
    - Not just for calm rooms—can add a gentle floral note to cleaning solutions.
    - Good if you dislike harsh or zesty smells.
6. **Thyme (Thymus vulgaris linalool chemotype)**
    - Some thyme oils can have strong cleansing qualities.
    - Must be used carefully because it can irritate skin.
    - Good in surface sprays for kitchen counters, but keep the dilution low.
7. **Pine (Pinus sylvestris)**
    - Classic "clean" scent.
    - Often associated with fresh forests.
    - Good for floors or bathrooms, but check if you like the strong pine aroma.

12.5 Safety Points for Using Essential Oils in Cleaning

1. **Ventilation**: Open windows or run a fan when cleaning with essential oils. Strong vapors can irritate your nose or eyes if the air is stagnant.
2. **Gloves**: If you handle concentrated oils or scrub surfaces for a long time, wear gloves to protect your hands.
3. **Surface Testing**: Some oils (especially citrus) can affect certain surfaces, like natural stone or some plastics. Test a small, hidden spot first.
4. **Label Your Bottles**: Always mark homemade cleaners with the ingredients and date. Keep out of reach of children and pets.
5. **Watch for Allergies**: If you or someone in the home has allergies, choose oils known to be gentler, or skip essential oils altogether.

12.6 All-Purpose Spray Recipes

An all-purpose cleaner can be used on many surfaces, like countertops, doorknobs, or sinks. However, avoid using vinegar-based cleaners on materials like marble or certain types of stone because vinegar's acidity can cause damage.

Simple Vinegar and Oil Spray

- 1 cup white vinegar
- 1 cup distilled water
- 10-15 drops of an essential oil (e.g., lemon or tea tree)
- Mix in a spray bottle. Shake before each use. Spray on surfaces and wipe with a cloth.

Mild Soap Spray

- 2 cups warm water
- 1 teaspoon liquid Castile soap
- 10 drops lavender or lemon essential oil
- Shake well in a spray bottle. Great for a quick wipe-down of counters or light messes.

Check a small area first if you worry about damaging the surface.

12.7 Kitchen Cleaning with Essential Oils

12.7.1 Countertops and Sinks

- **Lemon and Vinegar Mix**
    - 1 cup white vinegar
    - 1 cup water
    - 10 drops lemon essential oil
    - Spray and wipe with a cloth.
    - Rinse with plain water if needed, especially on delicate surfaces.
- **Baking Soda Paste**

- Mix baking soda with a little water until it forms a paste.
- Add 2 drops of tea tree essential oil.
- Scrub the sink gently, then rinse.
- Leaves a fresh look without strong chemicals.

12.7.2 Cutting Boards

- **Quick Freshen-Up**
    - Rub half a lemon on the board, let sit a few minutes, then rinse.
    - Optionally, add 1 drop of lemon or tea tree oil to the lemon half before rubbing.
    - Rinse well and air dry.

12.7.3 Garbage Disposal

- **Lemon and Ice**
    - Place a few small ice cubes in the disposal, add 2 drops lemon essential oil.
    - Turn on the disposal with running water.
    - The lemon scent can help reduce odors.
    - Always follow your disposal's manual for best practices.

12.8 Bathroom Cleaning with Essential Oils

Bathrooms can be prone to soap scum or mildew. Essential oils with stronger scents like tea tree, eucalyptus, or peppermint can help freshen up these areas.

12.8.1 Shower and Tub

- **Soap Scum Remover**
    - 1 cup white vinegar (warm it gently)
    - 1 cup dish soap (mild)
    - 10 drops eucalyptus essential oil
    - Mix in a spray bottle. Spray on shower walls and tub.
    - Let sit for 10–15 minutes, scrub, then rinse.

- **Baking Soda Scrub**
    - 1/2 cup baking soda
    - Enough water to form a thick paste
    - 2 drops tea tree oil
    - Spread on grimy areas, wait a few minutes, scrub, and rinse.

12.8.2 Toilet Bowl

- **Simple Toilet Cleaner**
    - 1/2 cup baking soda
    - 10 drops tea tree or lavender essential oil
    - Sprinkle into the toilet bowl, then pour in about 1/4 cup white vinegar. Let it fizz.
    - Scrub with a toilet brush and flush.

12.8.3 Mirrors and Glass

- **Glass Spray**
    - 1 cup distilled water
    - 1 cup white vinegar
    - 5 drops lemon or lavender oil
    - Spray on glass surfaces, wipe with a lint-free cloth or newspaper.
    - If streaks remain, reduce the amount of essential oil or skip it entirely. Some oils might slightly streak glass, so test first.

12.9 Floors and Carpets

12.9.1 Mopping Solutions

- **Vinegar Floor Cleaner**
    - 1 gallon warm water
    - 1/2 cup white vinegar
    - 10 drops lemon or pine essential oil
    - Use on tile or vinyl floors. Avoid wood floors if you are unsure about vinegar's effect.

- For wood floors, use less vinegar or a mild soap solution instead.
- **Soap-Based Mop Mix**
    - 1 gallon warm water
    - 1 tablespoon liquid Castile soap
    - 5 drops lavender oil
    - Mop as usual, and rinse with clean water if the floor feels soapy.

12.9.2 Carpet Refresh

- **Powder Deodorizer**
    - 1 cup baking soda
    - 10 drops lavender, peppermint, or lemon essential oil (choose just one scent, or a simple combination)
    - Mix well in a bowl, let it sit for an hour so the baking soda absorbs the oil.
    - Sprinkle lightly over the carpet, wait 15–20 minutes, then vacuum.
    - Helps absorb odors and leaves a mild scent.
- **Spot Cleaner**
    - Blot spills right away.
    - Use a mild soap and water mix first.
    - For a final fresh scent, place 1 drop of peppermint or lavender oil on a damp cloth and dab the area (test on hidden carpet corner first for discoloration).

12.10 Laundry Tips

Using essential oils in laundry can give clothes a light, natural scent. Keep in mind that the dryer's heat might reduce the aroma.

1. **Scented Wash**
    - Add 5–10 drops of an essential oil (like lavender or eucalyptus) to the washing machine's rinse cycle.
    - Or mix the drops with a carrier like a tablespoon of white vinegar before adding.

2. **Dryer Balls**
   - Place 2-3 drops of oil on wool dryer balls.
   - Toss them in the dryer with clothes.
   - This can help reduce static and add a gentle smell.
3. **Storage Sachets**
   - Put a few drops of lavender or cedarwood on a cotton ball or small cloth.
   - Place in your closet or drawers to keep clothes smelling fresh and discourage some pests like moths.

12.11 Dealing with Pests

Certain essential oils may help repel insects or rodents:

- **Peppermint**: Some people use cotton balls soaked with a few drops of peppermint oil around cracks or entry points to discourage mice or ants. Refresh every few days.
- **Cedarwood**: Often used in closets or chests to keep moths away from clothing.
- **Citronella or Lemongrass**: Known for repelling mosquitoes outside. But use caution if diffusing indoors, as the smell can be strong.

These methods might not remove a severe pest issue, but they can help as a mild deterrent.

12.12 Rare Ideas for Household Freshness

- **Car Interior**: Add 1-2 drops of your favorite oil to a cotton ball, place it under the seat. Avoid oils that might irritate skin if they spill.
- **Vacuum Cleaner**: Sprinkle a bit of scented baking soda on the floor and vacuum it up. The vacuum will release the aroma as you clean.
- **Trash Can Deodorizer**: Place a cotton ball with 2 drops of tea tree or lemon oil at the bottom of the bin (below the bag). Helps mask unpleasant smells.

- **Simple Room Spray**: Mix 1 cup of water, 1 tablespoon rubbing alcohol, and 10–15 drops of a favorite oil in a spray bottle. Shake and spray lightly in the air (not on surfaces that might stain).

12.13 Tips for Keeping it Simple

- **Do Not Overdo It**: A small amount of essential oil can go a long way. Using too many drops can create a strong haze.
- **Test Surfaces**: Especially with natural wood, granite, or marble, do a quick patch test. Vinegar and certain oils can dull or discolor some finishes.
- **Store Safely**: Homemade cleaners should be dated and stored away from children.
- **Shake Before Use**: Oil and water do not mix well, so always shake your spray bottles before each use.

12.14 Cost and Sourcing

Some people worry essential oils can be expensive. Indeed, certain oils like rose or jasmine can be costly. But for cleaning, you often only need cheaper oils such as lemon, tea tree, or peppermint. Buy from a reputable brand that provides clear labeling. You do not need the highest-grade oils for cleaning tasks, but do pick a pure essential oil instead of synthetic fragrance if you want the natural benefits.

12.15 Environmental Considerations

When using essential oils for cleaning, think about how they might impact the environment:

- **Sustainability**: Some oils come from plants that may be overharvested. Pick common, renewable plant oils when possible.

- **Waste Reduction**: Making your own cleaners can cut down on plastic waste if you reuse spray bottles.
- **Waterways**: Strong chemicals and large amounts of essential oils can end up in drains. Keep your usage moderate.

Try to find a balance that respects both your home environment and the outdoors.

12.16 When to Use Stronger Methods

Homemade cleaners with essential oils are good for everyday tidying. However, they might not be enough for deep disinfection in cases of serious illness, mold, or heavy grime. In such instances, you may need a specialized cleaner or bleach-based product. You can still use essential oils afterward to freshen the air, but do not rely solely on them for thorough sanitizing where pathogens might be an issue.

12.17 Avoiding Repetitive Scents

Using the same strong oil every day can make you grow tired of it. It could also lead to mild headaches if the smell is always around. Try rotating your oils:

- **Week 1**: Lemon-based cleaning.
- **Week 2**: Switch to lavender or peppermint.
- **Week 3**: Maybe pine or eucalyptus.

This keeps scents interesting and may reduce the chance of becoming overly sensitized to one particular aroma.

12.18 Protecting Pets and Children

When cleaning with essential oils, ensure kids and pets are not in the area if the room becomes heavily scented. Open windows or let the space air out before they enter. Dogs or cats may be more sensitive to certain scents, and birds especially can have a hard time with strong vapors. Always use caution and pay attention to signs of discomfort, such as sneezing or hiding.

12.19 Helpful Recipes Recap

Let's compile a few quick go-to recipes you can bookmark:

1. **All-Purpose Spray**
   - 1 cup water + 1 cup vinegar + 10 drops lemon = daily counter wipe-down.
2. **Bathroom Scrub**
   - 1/2 cup baking soda + 2 drops tea tree + water to form paste = tackle sinks and tubs.
3. **Glass Cleaner**
   - 1 cup water + 1 cup vinegar + 5 drops lavender = mirrors and windows.
4. **Floor Wash**
   - 1 gallon warm water + 1/2 cup vinegar + 10 drops pine = fresh-scented floors (not for delicate wood).
5. **Carpet Deodorizer**
   - 1 cup baking soda + 10 drops peppermint = sprinkle and vacuum.

Remember to adapt these recipes based on the surfaces in your home and your personal scent preferences. Always label and store safely.

12.20 Conclusion

Essential oils can be a pleasant addition to natural household cleaning routines. They supply fresh smells and can work hand-in-hand with basic items like vinegar, baking soda, and mild soap. By mixing just a few drops of oils such as lemon, tea tree, or lavender into homemade cleaners, you can maintain a home that smells light and clean without relying on strong synthetic chemicals.

At the same time, be mindful of safety. Keep solutions labeled and away from kids and pets. Open windows and do not overuse oils in small spaces. If you need heavy-duty disinfection, consider proven commercial products, then add a gentle essential oil blend later for a pleasing aroma. This balanced approach lets you enjoy a tidier home that also smells welcoming.

With these methods, you can refresh surfaces, carpets, and laundry. Over time, you might develop favorite blends that suit your household best. A mild lemon-vinegar spray, a lavender floor wash, or a peppermint baking soda mix—each can bring a gentle, natural feel to your cleaning tasks. By using essential oils with care, you can enjoy a cleaner home that aligns with a simpler, more natural lifestyle.

CHAPTER 13: Essential Oils for First Aid and Common Health Issues

13.1 Introduction to First Aid with Essential Oils

Every household handles small mishaps from time to time, like minor scrapes, insect bites, or mild skin irritations. Many people turn to over-the-counter ointments, but essential oils can also be part of a small first aid kit. They can provide a gentle option for cleaning, soothing discomfort, or reducing everyday issues. Of course, for major concerns, please seek medical help.

In this chapter, we will see how some essential oils can support mild first aid needs. We will also learn which oils match certain minor problems, the correct ways to use them, and when to step back and let a medical expert handle the situation. Keep in mind that children, older adults, and those with sensitive skin may need extra caution.

13.2 General Guidelines for First Aid with Oils

1. **Dilute Before Using**
    - Essential oils are strong. Even for a quick first aid response, most oils must be diluted in a carrier oil or water-based medium before touching the skin.
    - For spot applications (like on a small scrape), a 1–2% dilution is usually enough.
2. **Clean the Area**
    - Before applying oils to a cut or scrape, rinse the site with clean water. Remove any debris.
    - This makes sure no dirt gets trapped under an oily mixture.
3. **Patch Test if Time Allows**
    - If the situation is not urgent, do a tiny test on healthy skin first.
    - Wait a few minutes to see if there is a reaction.
4. **Stop if There Is Any Sign of Irritation**

- If the person experiences itching, redness, or burning, remove the oil by rinsing with mild soap and water.
- In some cases, wiping the area with a carrier oil (like sweet almond) can help reduce the intensity of the essential oil on the skin.

5. **Know When to Seek Help**
   - Essential oils are for mild problems. A deep cut, major burn, or serious allergic reaction needs proper medical care.
   - If an injury seems large, painful, or shows signs of infection, see a healthcare professional.

13.3 Essential Oils for Minor Cuts and Scrapes

13.3.1 Lavender (Lavandula angustifolia)

- **Why It Helps**: Lavender is known for its mild and soothing qualities. Some people use it to support clean skin and reduce redness.
- **How to Use**: Dilute 1–2 drops in a teaspoon (5 mL) of carrier oil. Gently dab on the clean scrape with a cotton swab.

13.3.2 Tea Tree (Melaleuca alternifolia)

- **Why It Helps**: Tea tree has been linked to properties that assist in limiting the spread of some unwanted microbes.
- **How to Use**: For a small cut, dilute 1 drop of tea tree in a teaspoon of carrier oil. Apply lightly around the cut. Do not place oils deep into the wound itself.

13.3.3 Chamomile (Roman or German)

- **Why It Helps**: Chamomile is gentle and often used for soothing irritated skin.
- **How to Use**: A 1% dilution is typically enough. This might be 1 drop in a teaspoon of carrier oil. Dab on the area to keep it calm.

For larger or deeper wounds, do not rely on essential oils alone. If bleeding is continuous or the wound looks serious, consult a doctor. Cleanliness and proper bandaging are also key.

13.4 Essential Oils for Minor Burns

Minor burns can happen while cooking or from brief contact with something hot. These are typically first-degree or small second-degree burns that cause redness or mild blistering. Anything severe (large blisters, charred skin, or a burn larger than a few inches) requires medical help.

1. **Cool Water First**
   - Immediately run the burn under cool (not ice-cold) water for several minutes. This helps lower skin temperature and reduce injury.
2. **Lavender**
   - A few people find that carefully diluted lavender may calm the stinging feeling.
   - Mix 1 drop of lavender in a teaspoon of aloe vera gel or clean carrier oil and gently apply a small amount.
3. **Aloe Vera + Essential Oil**
   - Many folks use aloe vera to soothe. You can add 1 drop of chamomile or lavender to a tablespoon (15 mL) of pure aloe gel.
   - Dab gently on the burned area, but do not rub.
4. **Observe**
   - Watch for signs of infection, like increasing redness, swelling, or pus.
   - If the burn does not improve or if pain is severe, see a healthcare professional.

13.5 Essential Oils for Bug Bites and Stings

Outdoor activities often lead to mosquito bites, bee stings, or contact with other insects. Essential oils might help reduce itch or minor swelling, but be aware that allergic reactions to stings can be dangerous and need quick medical care.

1. **Tea Tree**

- Commonly used for its cleansing effect on the skin.
- Dilute 1 drop in a teaspoon of carrier oil and dab on the bite or sting.
2. **Lavender**
    - Has a mild aroma that may reduce the urge to scratch.
    - 1-2 drops in a teaspoon of carrier oil, then apply carefully to the spot.
3. **Peppermint (Mentha x piperita)**
    - Some people find peppermint's cooling sensation helps with an itchy bite.
    - Must be used sparingly and in low dilution (like 0.5-1%) because it can irritate if too strong.

Important: If someone shows signs of a severe reaction (like trouble breathing or major swelling beyond the sting site), seek medical help quickly.

13.6 Essential Oils for Head Discomfort

Many people experience mild head tension or throbbing feelings sometimes. Essential oils will not replace medication for strong headaches, but they might ease mild ones.

1. **Peppermint**
    - Known for a cooling feeling that might help with mild head discomfort.
    - Dilute 1 drop in a teaspoon of carrier oil. Gently rub onto the temples or the back of the neck, avoiding the eyes.
2. **Lavender**
    - May calm the mind if tension is linked to stress.
    - Diffuse 2-3 drops or apply lightly (diluted) to the temples.
3. **Rosemary (Rosmarinus officinalis)**
    - Some people say rosemary can help with mental clarity, which may reduce mild head tension.
    - Keep dilution low (1%) to avoid skin sensitivity, especially near the face.

If head pain is severe, persistent, or accompanied by other symptoms (like fever or vision changes), talk to a healthcare professional.

13.7 Essential Oils for Mild Digestive Discomfort

Upset stomach, occasional cramps, or feeling queasy might happen due to stress, eating habits, or other minor causes. Essential oils can sometimes help with mild discomfort, but serious issues require a doctor's input.

1. **Peppermint**
    - Known for a fresh aroma that may help ease a feeling of queasiness.
    - People sometimes inhale peppermint from a tissue or a personal inhaler.
    - Topical use on the abdomen (diluted in a carrier oil) might also be soothing for mild cramps.
2. **Ginger (Zingiber officinale)**
    - Warm, spicy scent. Often linked to easing feelings of nausea.
    - Try 1 drop in a teaspoon of carrier oil, gently massage on the belly.
3. **Chamomile (Roman)**
    - Gentle and calming.
    - Could be diffused or used in a mild abdomen massage with a carrier oil.

Note: Ingestion of essential oils is usually discouraged unless guided by a qualified professional. A mild tea or a doctor-approved remedy may be safer for internal help.

13.8 Essential Oils for Mild Colds and Congestion

A minor cold can leave the nose stuffy and the head feeling heavy. Essential oils cannot cure a cold, but they might offer comfort by making breathing feel easier.

1. **Eucalyptus (Eucalyptus radiata or Eucalyptus smithii)**
    - Known for its cool, clearing scent.

- Add 2–3 drops to a bowl of hot water, lean over (not too close), cover your head with a towel, and inhale gently for a short time. Keep eyes closed and be careful with hot steam.
- Do not use eucalyptus globulus for very young kids; it can be too strong.
2. **Peppermint**
    - Another oil that can give a feeling of openness in the nasal area.
    - Similar steam method, but perhaps only 1 drop due to its strength.
3. **Tea Tree**
    - Some people include tea tree in steam blends for a fresh effect.
    - Use 1 drop or 2 drops in hot water. Inhale slowly with caution.

Also remember to rest, drink plenty of fluids, and watch for signs of more serious illness.

13.9 Sunburn and Skin Overexposure

A day outdoors might result in sunburn if we forget to apply sunscreen or stay in the shade. Mild sunburn causes redness and discomfort. Severe sunburn with blisters, chills, or large areas of damaged skin needs medical attention.

1. **Cool the Area**
    - Rinse with cool water or place a cold compress on the affected spots.
2. **Aloe Vera Gel + Essential Oils**
    - Mix 2 drops of lavender or chamomile in 1 tablespoon (15 mL) of pure aloe vera gel.
    - Gently dab on the sunburned skin, do not rub too hard.
3. **Hydrate**
    - Drink extra water and rest.
    - Keep an eye on any sign of serious sun damage.

13.10 Muscle Aches and Stiffness

After exercise, manual labor, or sleeping in a bad position, muscles might feel sore or stiff. Essential oils can enhance a relaxing massage or warm compress.

1. **Lavender**
   - A top choice for muscle tension. It can help the person feel calmer overall.
   - Add 3 drops to 1 tablespoon (15 mL) of carrier oil and gently massage the sore area.
2. **Marjoram (Origanum majorana)**
   - Known for its warming effect. May be used for minor aches.
   - Keep dilution around 1-2% to avoid irritation.
3. **Rosemary**
   - Stimulating scent that some people find comforting on stiff muscles.
   - A warm compress: Fill a bowl with warm water, add 2 drops rosemary, soak a cloth, and apply to the area.

If aches are severe, repeated, or get worse, see a doctor.

13.11 Supporting Mild Stress and Nervous Feelings

Small first aid needs are not always physical; sometimes they relate to a sudden wave of nervousness or mild panic. We covered stress in a previous chapter, but here are quick tips:

- **Inhaler or Tissue Method**: Put 1-2 drops of lavender or chamomile on a tissue, inhale gently to settle nerves.
- **Simple Hand Massage**: Dilute a calming oil in carrier oil, gently rub hands or temples.
- **Focus on Breathing**: Combine the aroma with slow, steady breaths.

Seek professional help if the person experiences ongoing anxiety or panic attacks that disrupt daily life.

13.12 Rare Insights and Handy Tips

1. **Cotton Swab or Cotton Ball**: This can help apply oils precisely to a small area, like a bug bite or cut, without over-applying.
2. **Roller Bottles**: Preparing a few low-dilution roller blends for first aid is convenient. Label them clearly (for cuts, bites, or head tension).
3. **Chilled Aloe Gel**: Storing aloe gel in the fridge can give extra cooling relief when mixed with essential oils for burns or sunburn.
4. **Allergy or Sensitivity Warning**: Even if an oil is "safe" for many people, some individuals can still react negatively. Always stay alert.
5. **Check Shelf Life**: Old or oxidized oils can irritate the skin more. Replace them if they have been open for too long or smell off.

13.13 When Essential Oils Are Not Enough

- **Serious Wounds**: Deep or heavily bleeding cuts, or any wound with debris that cannot be cleaned easily, need medical attention.
- **Major Burns**: Large blisters, white or charred skin, or burned areas on the face, hands, feet, or groin require urgent care.
- **Allergic Reactions**: Swelling of the face, lips, or throat, trouble breathing, or widespread hives demand immediate help.
- **Extreme Pain**: If pain is out of proportion to a simple first aid scenario, see a professional.

Essential oils can be supportive, but they do not replace a thorough medical evaluation when needed.

13.14 Building a Basic Essential Oil First Aid Kit

1. **Tea Tree Oil**: Good for cleaning small cuts or insect bites.
2. **Lavender Oil**: Soothing for burns, bites, mild stress, or small headaches.
3. **Chamomile Oil**: Gentle choice for children or people with sensitive skin.

4. **Peppermint Oil**: Cooling effect for head tension or mild muscle aches (use carefully).
5. **Carrier Oil**: A small bottle of fractionated coconut, sweet almond, or jojoba is important.
6. **Aloe Vera Gel**: For burns and sunburn relief, plus easy mixing with certain oils.
7. **Bandaids, Gauze, Tweezers**: Essential oils alone are not enough. Basic first aid items help complete the kit.
8. **Labels and Instructions**: Mark each oil with the name and any warning. Keep instructions for safe dilution rates on hand.

13.15 Blending Examples for Quick Application

Minor Cut Blend

- 1 drop tea tree + 1 drop lavender in 2 teaspoons (10 mL) carrier oil.
- Store in a small bottle. Use a cotton swab on clean minor cuts.

Itch-Soothing Blend

- 1 drop peppermint + 2 drops lavender in 2 teaspoons (10 mL) carrier oil.
- Dab on insect bites or mild itchy spots.

Head Comfort Roller

- 1 drop peppermint + 2 drops lavender in 1 tablespoon (15 mL) carrier oil.
- Put in a roller bottle, apply to temples (avoid eyes) or back of neck.

13.16 Dealing with Allergic Contact

Sometimes, essential oils can be part of the problem if someone has an allergy. It is also possible that a person might be allergic to a plant family.

For example, those allergic to ragweed might react to chamomile. In these cases:

1. **Remove the Oil**
   - Wipe the area with carrier oil or wash with mild soap and water.
2. **Apply Cool Compress**
   - A cloth soaked in cool water can lessen redness or itching.
3. **Observe for Larger Reaction**
   - If it worsens, see a healthcare provider.

13.17 Essential Oils and Pets in Emergencies

Sometimes, people use essential oils to help pets with small problems. But be careful: animals can react differently than humans. For example, tea tree can be toxic to some pets if used incorrectly. Consult a veterinarian with knowledge of essential oils before applying them to pets. In cases of pet emergencies, go to a vet right away rather than relying on oils.

13.18 Emergencies While Traveling

When traveling, keep a small first aid bag handy. You can pack:

- **Travel-Sized Carrier Oil**
- **A Few Multi-Purpose Oils** (like lavender or tea tree in 5 mL bottles)
- **Basic Items**: Bandages, small scissors, tweezers, alcohol wipes

Be sure to comply with airline rules about liquids. Also, keep in mind how the body might react to essential oils in different climates or altitudes. Watch out for strong sun when using oils like lemon or bergamot on skin. They can cause photosensitivity.

13.19 Myths About Essential Oils in First Aid

- **Myth: Neat Application Is Always Fine**
  - Some people say you can use oils straight from the bottle on wounds. This can be very irritating, especially with strong oils. Dilution is safer.
- **Myth: Replacing All Modern Care**
  - While oils can help in mild cases, they do not replace antibiotics for severe infections or other needed treatments.
- **Myth: All Burns Need Lavender**
  - Some burns do not respond well to oils if they are deep or severe. Always cool with water first and assess the seriousness.
- **Myth: More Drops = Faster Healing**
  - In fact, more drops can cause irritation. Less can often be more.

13.20 Conclusion

Essential oils can provide gentle support for small, everyday mishaps like minor cuts, insect bites, or mild sunburn. They can also soothe simple head tensions or muscle aches. With correct dilution and careful application, they may be a helpful addition to a basic first aid approach.

However, they have limits. They do not replace professional medical care when problems are serious. Always pay attention to signs that an injury or illness needs expert treatment. Keep in mind that every person reacts differently to oils. What calms one person might irritate another. By knowing a few core oils (lavender, tea tree, chamomile, peppermint) and safe ways to use them, you can prepare a small "natural first aid" kit. Combine this with standard items and knowledge of when to seek professional help, and you will have a balanced plan for minor health issues.

CHAPTER 14: Essential Oils and Aromatherapy

14.1 Introduction to Aromatherapy

Aromatherapy is a practice that uses scents from essential oils to support well-being. People have inhaled plant aromas for centuries, whether through burnt resins, fresh herbs, or distilled oils. Modern aromatherapy often involves diffusers, inhalers, massages, or baths to bring these natural aromas into daily routines.

In this chapter, we will look at the fundamentals of aromatherapy, how scents can affect emotions or certain body functions, and ways to incorporate these ideas safely into your life. The goal is to help you understand the basics of the practice and choose methods that fit your lifestyle.

14.2 The Science Behind Aromatherapy

When you inhale an essential oil, scent molecules interact with smell receptors in your nose. These receptors send signals to the limbic system, a part of the brain tied to emotions and memories. This can explain why certain scents remind you of events or feelings. Some scents may help you feel calmer or more upbeat.

However, not everyone responds to scents in the same way. Culture, personal history, and genetics can shape how you experience an aroma. Also, while some small studies suggest certain oils can shift mood or support relaxation, large-scale research is still growing. Aromatherapy often acts as a comforting addition rather than a guaranteed cure.

14.3 Popular Aromatherapy Methods

1. **Diffusion**
    - A common approach that spreads scent into the air.

- Can be done with an electric diffuser or a simple bowl of warm water.
- Choose a safe number of drops (3–6) for a moderate-sized room.

2. **Inhaler Sticks**
   - Small, portable tubes with a wick inside.
   - You add essential oils onto the wick, close it, and sniff when needed.
   - Useful for quick relief in stressful moments.
3. **Steam Inhalation**
   - A bowl of hot water with a few drops of essential oil.
   - You lean over, drape a towel around your head, and breathe slowly.
   - Ideal for helping with stuffy noses (use caution with kids or those sensitive to strong scents).
4. **Topical Use**
   - Aromatherapy massages or roller bottles.
   - The scent is still inhaled while the oil is applied to the skin.
   - Always dilute to avoid irritation.
5. **Room Sprays**
   - Mix water, a little alcohol (like vodka or rubbing alcohol), and essential oils in a spray bottle.
   - Shake and spritz in the air or on fabrics (test first).
   - Quick way to freshen a space.

14.4 Choosing the Right Oils for Aromatherapy

Selecting an oil often depends on your goals:

- **Calm and Relaxation**: Lavender, chamomile, cedarwood
- **Uplifting**: Citrus oils (lemon, orange, bergamot), peppermint
- **Focus**: Rosemary, basil, lemon
- **Emotional Support**: Rose, ylang ylang, frankincense

You can pick single oils or blend a few to create a layered aroma. Many folks enjoy balancing top notes (citrus, mint) with middle notes (florals, herbs) and base notes (woods, resins). Each note evaporates at a different rate, shaping how the scent unfolds.

14.5 Essential Tools for Aromatherapy

1. **Diffuser**: Electric diffusers come with a small water reservoir. You add a few drops of oil, and the device disperses the aroma.
2. **Inhaler Blanks**: Often sold in bulk, they are inexpensive tubes that let you create personal aromatherapy sticks.
3. **Carrier Oils**: For massages, you need a base oil like jojoba, sweet almond, or fractionated coconut.
4. **Dark Glass Bottles**: Useful for storing custom blends.
5. **Labels**: Always label your blends with ingredients and the date.

14.6 Safety in Aromatherapy

Though aromatherapy can seem simple, there are safety rules:

- **Ventilation**: Do not overfill the air with strong aromas. Open a window or door to keep fresh air flowing.
- **Short Sessions**: Diffuse for about 15–30 minutes at a time, then take a break.
- **Watch for Sensitivities**: Some people get headaches from scents or have allergic reactions. Stop if you notice discomfort.
- **Children and Pets**: Use less oil around them, and choose gentle scents like lavender.
- **Medical Conditions**: If someone has asthma or breathing issues, test carefully. Strong scents might trigger episodes.

14.7 Using Aromatherapy for Emotional Wellness

Aromatherapy often centers on emotional well-being:

1. **Stress Relief**
    - Diffuse lavender, bergamot, or chamomile in the evening.
    - Practice slow breathing while enjoying the scent.

2. **Mood Lifting**
   - Citrus oils can bring a fresh, positive atmosphere.
   - Start the morning with a short diffusion of sweet orange or grapefruit.
3. **Memory Support**
   - Rosemary has been tied (in some small studies) to alertness.
   - Try an inhaler stick before studying or reading, but keep it mild to avoid overwhelming the senses.
4. **Grief or Sadness**
   - Rose or frankincense might offer comfort for some.
   - Softly diffused or worn in a personal inhaler.

Remember, these are supportive practices, not replacements for therapy or counseling when facing deeper emotional challenges.

14.8 Aromatherapy and the Body

While inhalation is the main focus, some people believe that scents can have secondary effects on the body. For instance:

- **Breathing**: Oils like eucalyptus, peppermint, or pine can make airways feel more open.
- **Skin**: Aromatherapy massage (with safe dilution) can relax muscles and ease tension.
- **Sleep**: A bedroom diffuser with lavender or chamomile might help set a restful mood.

However, each body is unique. Always pay attention to how you feel and adjust if something is unpleasant.

14.9 Rare Tips for Deepening Aromatherapy

1. **Scent Journal**
   - Write down which oils you used, how you felt, and any changes you noticed.
   - Over time, you might see patterns, like which oil really helps you relax on stressful days.

2. **Pair with Relaxation Activities**
   - Use soft music or read a calming book while inhaling mild scents.
   - This can amplify the soothing effect.
3. **Scent Rotation**
   - If you smell the same oil every day, your brain might start ignoring it.
   - Switch oils or take a few days off to keep the effect fresh.
4. **Scent Anchoring**
   - Choose a specific oil for a certain activity, like lemon for studying or lavender for bedtime.
   - Over time, your brain may link that aroma with the activity, making it easier to focus or rest.

14.10 Creating Custom Aromatherapy Blends

1. **Balance Notes**
   - Combine top, middle, and base notes. For example:
     - Top: Lemon or bergamot
     - Middle: Lavender or geranium
     - Base: Cedarwood or frankincense
   - A simple ratio is 3 drops top : 2 drops middle : 1 drop base, but you can adjust.
2. **Test in Small Batches**
   - Use a small bottle or even a shot glass to blend a few drops at a time.
   - Wave it under your nose, see if you like it. Tweak as needed.
3. **Let It Rest**
   - Some blends change character after a day or two. This resting time helps the scents mix.
   - Re-sniff after 24 hours and note the aroma.
4. **Dilute for Use**
   - If you plan to apply to skin, remember to add carrier oil. For diffusion, you can keep it as a pure essential oil mix but use fewer drops in the diffuser.

14.11 Aromatherapy Baths and Foot Soaks

Baths can be a nice way to combine warmth and scent:

1. **Bath Safety**
    - Essential oils do not mix well with water alone. They float on the surface and can cling to skin in concentrated spots.
    - Mix the oil with a carrier (like a tablespoon of unscented liquid soap or a carrier oil) before adding to the bath.
2. **Foot Soaks**
    - A basin of warm water, plus 2-3 drops of an oil like peppermint or lavender, can soothe tired feet.
    - Test the temperature, especially for older adults or those with limited sensation in their feet.
3. **Quantity**
    - For a full bath, 5-8 drops of essential oil (properly dispersed) is often enough.
    - For a foot soak, 2-3 drops is plenty.

14.12 Aromatherapy Massage Basics

Aromatherapy massages combine the effects of gentle touch with the aromas of oils:

1. **Choose a Carrier Oil**
    - Sweet almond, jojoba, or fractionated coconut are common.
    - Aim for a dilution of about 1-2% for an adult. That might be 2-3 drops of essential oil per tablespoon (15 mL) of carrier.
2. **Gentle Strokes**
    - Massage helps relax muscles and improves circulation.
    - The person also inhales the scent, offering a combined benefit.
3. **Check for Preferences**
    - Some people dislike certain smells. Always ask first.
    - Keep a towel handy in case the aroma becomes overwhelming and you need to wipe off the oil.
4. **Time and Setting**

- A quiet, warm room and soothing background music can enhance the experience.

14.13 Cultural Roots of Aromatherapy

Across the world, different cultures used aromatic plants in ceremonies, health practices, or daily life:

- **Egyptians**: Known for using fragrant resins and oils in rituals.
- **Traditional Chinese Practices**: Herbs and aromatic extracts appear in many historic texts.
- **Ayurveda (India)**: Incorporates plant-based oils in massages and wellness methods.
- **Greek and Roman Traditions**: Baths and body oils infused with fragrances were popular.

Modern aromatherapy draws on many of these traditions but adapts them with newer extraction techniques and scientific knowledge.

14.14 Emotional Support Through Aromatherapy

We discussed mood and essential oils in an earlier chapter, but it fits within aromatherapy's scope:

- **Diffusing for Calm Moods**
    - A small bedroom diffuser with 2 drops of lavender and 1 drop of cedarwood can create a calm evening vibe.
- **Inhalers for Stressful Moments**
    - Keep a personal stick with a calming blend (lavender + chamomile) in your pocket or purse.
- **Workplace Uplift**
    - If permitted, use a fan diffuser with sweet orange or lemon to keep the room fresh and positive.

Remember that not everyone around you will enjoy or tolerate scents, so consider others if you share the space.

14.15 Aromatherapy and Meditation

Some people pair aromatherapy with mindfulness or meditation to improve focus or relaxation:

1. **Select a Gentle Oil**
    - Frankincense is often used for spiritual or meditative practices.
    - Sandalwood is another option, but it can be expensive.
2. **Create a Quiet Space**
    - Diffuse 2–3 drops or light a candle-based diffuser.
    - Sit or lie down, close your eyes, and pay attention to the breath and the subtle scent.
3. **Set a Time Limit**
    - Even 5–10 minutes can be beneficial.
    - Keep the diffuser on a low setting or turn it off after a short while.

14.16 Aromatherapy for Group Settings

1. **Workshops or Classes**
    - Some yoga or art classes use mild diffusion of lavender or citrus to create a calm environment.
    - Always ask participants first if they have allergies or aversions.
2. **Hospitals or Care Homes**
    - In certain places, gentle aromatherapy is used for relaxation.
    - Must be done under guidelines to ensure it does not affect patients with breathing issues.
3. **Family Gatherings**
    - A simple diffuser with sweet orange or peppermint might freshen the room.
    - Keep the level subtle so it does not overpower conversation or meals.

14.17 Handling Challenges in Aromatherapy

- **Scent Overload**: Too many drops or multiple diffusers in a small space can cause headaches. Use fewer drops and take breaks.
- **Conflicting Aromas**: Burning scented candles, cooking food, and diffusing oils at the same time can clash. Choose one aroma source.
- **Storage**: Keep oils in a dark, cool place. Label each bottle with the purchase date.
- **Oxidized Oils**: Old oils, especially citrus, may develop a sharp or rancid smell. If in doubt, discard.

14.18 Rare Tips to Boost Aromatherapy at Home

1. **Scented Sachets**
   - Put a few drops of an essential oil on dried flowers or cotton, then place in small fabric bags.
   - Stash these in drawers, closets, or near the pillow (but not directly on fabric that might stain).
2. **Aroma Stones**
   - Small porous stones that can hold a few drops of oil.
   - Good for desks or places where you do not want a powered diffuser.
3. **Cotton Ball Trick**
   - If you do not have a diffuser, drip 1–2 drops on a cotton ball and place it in a cup or small dish.
   - The scent will diffuse slowly.
4. **Car Aromatherapy**
   - Some people use vent clips designed for essential oils.
   - Keep it mild to avoid distracting yourself while driving.

14.19 Debunking Aromatherapy Myths

- **Myth: Aromatherapy Fixes All Health Issues**
   - Aromatherapy can support mood or mild discomfort, but it is not a cure-all. Seek a doctor for serious concerns.

- **Myth: More Scent = Better Results**
  - Using too many drops at once can irritate. Small amounts are often enough.
- **Myth: All Oils Are Good for Everyone**
  - Each person has different sensitivities. Some oils might not be suitable if you have a specific allergy or condition.
- **Myth: Aromatherapy Is Only for Relaxation**
  - While it is well known for calm feelings, certain oils (like peppermint or rosemary) can help you feel more alert.

14.20 Conclusion

Aromatherapy is about using the power of scent to support comfort, mood, and sometimes mild physical relief. Whether you are diffusing lavender before bedtime, applying a ginger compress for tension, or simply using an uplifting citrus aroma while doing chores, the main goal is to enhance well-being in a gentle way.

By combining a basic understanding of the sense of smell with knowledge of different oils, you can tailor aromatherapy to your preferences. Keep safety in mind, especially around children, older adults, and pets. Ventilate your spaces, use moderate amounts of oil, and observe how you feel.

Over time, you may discover blends or single oils that become favorites for relaxation, focus, or emotional support. Aromatherapy can be as simple as inhaling a drop on a cotton ball or as involved as creating layered blends for specific aims. In any case, the key is mindful use and respect for the power of scent. When practiced with care, aromatherapy can add small, pleasant moments to daily life and serve as a handy tool for simple well-being.

CHAPTER 15: Essential Oils in Culinary Applications

15.1 Introduction to Cooking with Essential Oils

Many people know that essential oils can be used for things like aromatherapy, skin care, or household cleaning. But they may be surprised to hear that some essential oils can also be included in cooking. In some cases, essential oils come from the same herbs or spices already used in recipes. Think about basil, oregano, or lemon. The idea is that you can get very strong flavor from just a drop or two of an essential oil.

However, not all essential oils are safe to eat, and not all cooking methods will work well with them. There are special tips, safety factors, and flavor guidelines to keep in mind. This chapter will guide you through how to choose oils, how to use small amounts, and what to avoid. Remember, if you have doubts about any oil, it is best to double-check with a reliable source before using it in your meal.

15.2 Understanding Culinary-Grade Essential Oils

In some places, certain brands label their essential oils as "food safe" or "culinary grade." That means they have been tested or approved for limited use in foods, following local regulations. But there is no single worldwide standard. Each country can have its own rules about which oils are allowed in foods.

1. **Purity**: The oil must not have synthetic additives. You do not want extra chemicals that are not safe for eating.
2. **Proper Labeling**: If an oil says "not for internal use," do not cook with it.
3. **Botanical Name**: Check the exact type of plant. For example, sweet basil (*Ocimum basilicum*) is more common in cooking. Another variety might taste different or have unwanted effects.

4. **Concentration**: Even if an oil is pure, it is extremely potent. You only need a tiny amount, usually measured in drops.

For instance, lemon essential oil might come from the same type of lemon peel you use to flavor desserts or marinades. However, the oil is far more concentrated than lemon juice or zest, so a single drop can affect the entire dish.

15.3 Safety Precautions

1. **Dilution in a Carrier**: Many experts recommend that if you plan to add an essential oil to a recipe, first mix it into a carrier ingredient (like olive oil, melted butter, or honey) rather than putting drops straight into your pot. This helps spread out the oil so that you do not get a "hot spot" of intense flavor.
2. **Low Heat or No Heat**: Some essential oils lose their flavor or can change character if you heat them too much. Others might become bitter. Often, it is best to add the oil near the end of cooking or use it in unheated foods like dressings, dips, or no-bake sweets.
3. **Check for Personal Reactions**: Even if the oil is labeled food safe, some people might have a sensitivity or allergy. Start small, try a small sample, and see if your body is okay with it.
4. **Pregnancy and Children**: Always be extra careful. Young children may be more sensitive to strong substances. People who are pregnant might want to avoid certain oils entirely. If you have any concerns, ask a healthcare professional.
5. **No Overuse**: A single drop can be enough for an entire recipe, especially for strong oils like oregano or thyme. Overdoing it can ruin the meal and possibly upset your stomach.

15.4 Best Essential Oils for Cooking

Below are oils that people commonly use in food, but remember to check local guidelines:

1. **Citrus Oils** (e.g., lemon, lime, sweet orange)
    - Offer a bright flavor for baked goods, marinades, or salad dressings.
    - One drop often equals about a teaspoon of zest, though this can vary.
    - Add them at the end of cooking or in cold recipes to keep the fresh aroma.
2. **Herb Oils** (e.g., basil, oregano, thyme, rosemary)
    - Give a strong herbal note, like using dried herbs but more powerful.
    - Common in pasta sauces, soups, or roasted dishes.
    - A tiny drop can replace a teaspoon or more of the dried herb, though you might still use both for complexity.
3. **Peppermint Oil**
    - Used in desserts, especially chocolate-related ones, or in some sweet drinks.
    - Very strong, so often a toothpick dip (touching the toothpick to the oil, then swirling in the recipe) might be enough rather than a full drop.
4. **Ginger Oil**
    - Adds a warm, spicy note to stir-fries, baked goods, or beverages.
    - Use sparingly, as it can become overwhelming quickly.
5. **Lavender Oil**
    - Less common, but it can lend a floral taste to certain cookies, ice creams, or lemonades.
    - Must be a food-safe variety, and only a tiny amount. Overuse can make your dish taste like soap.

15.5 Practical Ways to Use Essential Oils in the Kitchen

1. **Dressings and Sauces**
    - Combine olive oil, vinegar or lemon juice, a bit of honey or mustard, and a drop of an essential oil like basil or lemon.
    - Shake well and taste. Adjust by adding more base ingredients if the flavor is too strong.
2. **Seasoned Oils**

- In a small glass bottle, add a carrier oil (like extra virgin olive oil). Stir in 1-2 drops of an herb essential oil.
- Let it sit for a day and then drizzle over bread, salads, or pasta. If it is too strong, dilute it further with plain oil.

3. **Bakery Items**
   - For cookies or cakes, you might add 1 drop of a citrus oil or peppermint to the batter. Mix thoroughly.
   - Be mindful that heat can change the flavor, so do a test batch if possible.

4. **No-Bake Treats**
   - Energy balls, raw cheesecakes, or homemade fudge might benefit from a single drop of a matching oil (like peppermint for a chocolate fudge).
   - Because these treats are not baked, the full flavor of the oil will remain. Start with half a drop if you can, or use the toothpick method.

5. **Marinades**
   - For meat or vegetables, blend your usual marinade (oil, acid like vinegar or lemon juice, spices) and add a drop of thyme or oregano essential oil.
   - Let the flavors mingle, then taste before soaking your food. You can add more salt, sugar, or other spices to balance out the strength of the oil.

15.6 Understanding Flavor Balance

Cooking with essential oils is about balance. A meal needs a mix of salty, sweet, sour, bitter, and possibly spicy flavors to feel complete. Essential oils, especially herbal or citrus ones, often fill the "aromatic" role. They can give a strong top note that brightens or sharpens the overall taste.

- **Pairing Citrus with Herbs**: A little lemon oil can bring out the bright side of rosemary or thyme in a roasted dish.
- **Combining Sweet and Minty**: Peppermint or spearmint oil in a dessert can cut through the richness of chocolate or cream.
- **Salt or Sugar Adjustments**: If your dish tastes too sharp after adding an essential oil, a bit of salt or sweetness might round it out.

- **Taste As You Go**: You can add more oil if it is too weak, but removing it once it is in your dish is impossible. So go slowly.

15.7 Conversion Tips

Recipes might call for fresh herbs, dried herbs, or zest. If you want to use essential oils instead, you need a rough conversion idea:

- **Zest of 1 Lemon** ≈ 1/8 to 1/4 teaspoon of lemon zest powder ≈ 1 drop of lemon essential oil (but depends on the brand).
- **1 Teaspoon Dried Herb** (like oregano) ≈ 1 drop essential oil. In many cases, half a drop or a toothpick swirl might be enough.

These are only approximations. Each brand of oil can differ. The best practice is to start small and add more if needed.

15.8 Using Essential Oils in Beverages

1. **Infused Water**
    - If you like flavored water, you could add 1 drop of lemon or grapefruit oil to a large pitcher. Stir well.
    - Watch out for oils that might irritate the lips if they collect on the surface. Shake or stir each time.
    - Some people prefer adding a few slices of real fruit as well to keep the flavor gentle.
2. **Teas and Hot Drinks**
    - You can swirl a toothpick with peppermint oil in a mug of hot chocolate or tea.
    - Heating can sometimes weaken or change the oil's taste, so add it near the end, just before drinking.
3. **Cocktails or Mocktails**
    - Mix a drop of lime oil into a pitcher with sweeteners, soda water, or fruit juices for a bright flavor.
    - Stir or shake well to distribute the oil.

- Garnish with fresh herbs or fruit slices to reinforce the aroma.
4. **Smoothies**
    - If you make a fruit smoothie, one drop of an essential oil like orange or spearmint might add a fun twist.
    - Blend thoroughly to avoid pockets of strong oil.

15.9 Special Considerations for Different Diets

- **Vegetarian or Vegan**: Using essential oils can be an easy way to add flavor to plant-based foods without introducing any animal products, as long as the oil itself does not use animal-derived additives (rare, but worth checking).
- **Gluten-Free**: Essential oils usually have no gluten, so they can spice up a gluten-free dish.
- **Low-Sodium**: Instead of salt, you might rely on flavorful oils like basil or oregano to give depth to a meal.
- **Sugar-Free**: Citrus or mint oils can offer bright tastes without adding any sugar.

When cooking for those with dietary restrictions, ensure the entire dish meets their needs, not just the flavoring.

15.10 Common Mistakes

1. **Using Oils That Are Not Food Safe**: Double-check the label or consult a trusted source. Some oils might have contaminants or are simply not meant to be eaten.
2. **Overuse**: One or two drops might be enough for a large batch of food. Adding more can make the meal taste medicinal or bitter.
3. **Poor Mixing**: Dropping oil into a hot pan without stirring or using a carrier can lead to uneven flavors.
4. **Ignoring Best-By Dates**: Citrus oils can oxidize over time, changing in taste. Old oils might taste off.

5. **Incorrect Storage**: Keep oils in a cool, dark place so they do not degrade. Heat and light can reduce flavor quality.

15.11 Rare Tips and Tricks

- **Toothpick Swirl Method**: If a drop is still too strong, dip a clean toothpick into the essential oil bottle, then swirl it into your dish. This transfers a fraction of a drop. It is handy for peppermint, oregano, or thyme.
- **Brightening Up Leftovers**: A single drop of lemon oil in a leftover soup or stew can lift the flavor. Add it when reheating, but not boiling.
- **Chocolate Pairings**: Peppermint, orange, and sometimes a tiny amount of lavender oil can pair well with chocolate. Do a small test batch first.
- **Flavoring Sea Salt or Sugar**: You can put a drop or two of an oil in a jar of sugar or salt, seal it, and let it absorb for a week. Then use that salt or sugar in recipes for a subtle infused taste.

15.12 Example Recipes

15.12.1 Lemon Herb Dressing

- **Ingredients**:
    1. 1/4 cup extra virgin olive oil
    2. 2 tablespoons white wine vinegar (or apple cider vinegar)
    3. 1 teaspoon Dijon mustard (optional)
    4. 1 drop lemon essential oil (food safe)
    5. 1 drop oregano or basil essential oil (optional, and if you do use it, skip dried oregano)
    6. Pinch of salt and pepper
- **Method**:
    1. In a small bowl or mason jar, whisk together the oil, vinegar, and mustard.

2. Dip a toothpick in the oregano oil (if using) and swirl it into the mixture. Add 1 drop of lemon oil.
3. Taste and adjust salt, pepper, or vinegar. If the flavor is too strong, add more olive oil.
4. Drizzle over salads or use as a marinade.

15.12.2 Chocolate Mint Fudge

- **Ingredients**:
    1. 1 can (14 oz) sweetened condensed milk
    2. 3 cups semi-sweet chocolate chips
    3. 1 drop peppermint essential oil (food safe)
    4. Pinch of salt
- **Method**:
    1. In a saucepan, warm the condensed milk over low heat.
    2. Add chocolate chips and stir until melted and smooth.
    3. Remove from heat. Wait a bit for it to cool slightly (so the oil won't evaporate too quickly).
    4. Stir in 1 drop of peppermint oil.
    5. Pour into a lined 8x8-inch pan. Let cool and set in the fridge.
    6. Cut into squares. If the mint flavor is too faint, next time try the toothpick swirl with two or more swirls.

15.12.3 Orange Smoothie

- **Ingredients**:
    1. 1 cup orange juice
    2. 1/2 cup plain yogurt (or a non-dairy alternative)
    3. 1 banana
    4. 1 drop sweet orange essential oil (food safe)
    5. Ice cubes (optional)
- **Method**:
    1. Combine orange juice, yogurt, banana, and ice in a blender.
    2. Blend until smooth.
    3. Pause and add 1 drop of orange oil. Blend again briefly.
    4. Taste. Add honey if needed or more banana for sweetness.

15.13 Hosting and Serving Suggestions

- **Label Foods**: If you are hosting a party, let guests know you used an essential oil in a dish. Some might have sensitivities or prefer to know what they are eating.
- **Small Bites**: Try out essential oil recipes in small servings (like mini cupcakes or a small batch of dips) to see if you like the result.
- **Complementary Fresh Garnishes**: If you made a lemon-thyme dish with essential oils, garnish with fresh thyme leaves or lemon zest so guests know the main flavor.
- **Drinks Station**: Place a sign next to your water pitcher or punch bowl if you used essential oils there. Include real fruit slices for an extra visual clue.

15.14 Possible Side Effects or Concerns

Even if an oil is labeled safe for cooking, there can be concerns:

1. **Digestive Upset**: Very strong or hot oils (like clove, cinnamon, or oregano) might irritate the stomach if you use too much.
2. **Taste Bud Overwhelm**: Some people just might not enjoy the powerful flavor.
3. **Medication Interactions**: If you are on certain meds, even small amounts of some oils could interfere. Check with a healthcare provider if unsure.
4. **Chemical Changes with Heat**: High heat cooking (like frying) can alter the oil's compounds. Some might produce off-tastes or new substances. It is usually safer to add these oils at a lower temperature stage or after removing the pan from direct heat.

15.15 Frequently Asked Questions

1. **Can I use any essential oil in my cupboard for cooking?**
    - No, only use ones that are labeled or confirmed as safe for culinary use.

2. **What if I accidentally add too many drops?**
   - If your recipe becomes too strong, you may try increasing other ingredients to dilute the flavor. In some cases, you might have to discard the dish.
3. **Should I use plastic or glass mixing bowls?**
   - Glass or stainless steel is usually better. Essential oils can damage some plastics or retain odors.
4. **How do I store essential oils for cooking?**
   - In a cool, dark place, tightly sealed. Keep away from heat and direct sunlight. And note the best-by date.
5. **Is it okay to ingest the oil directly on the tongue?**
   - Generally no. Essential oils are very potent and can irritate the mouth or throat. Always mix them in food or a carrier.

15.16 Closing Thoughts on Culinary Essential Oils

Cooking with essential oils can open new flavor doors. A dash of lemon or basil oil can transform simple dishes. But it is not something to do without thought. You need to ensure the oils are truly safe, handle them with caution, and measure carefully.

If you have never tried it before, start with a single oil, like lemon or peppermint, and see how it fits in one recipe. Keep track of what you learn. Over time, you may find a few favorite pairings—maybe an oregano oil marinade or a peppermint-laced dessert.

If you decide to include essential oils more often, keep searching for proven recipes or tips from reliable sources. Combine the best of your kitchen instincts with a gentle approach to these powerful plant extracts. That way, you will enjoy the flavors without going overboard.

CHAPTER 16: Advanced Blending Techniques

16.1 Introduction to Advanced Blending

Earlier chapters described simple ways to combine essential oils for everyday uses, such as diffuser blends or basic skincare mixes. This chapter goes further by exploring more detailed blending methods. Advanced blending is about crafting harmonious aromas or specialized mixtures for certain goals—like a unique perfume or a precise therapy blend for relaxation.

People who get into advanced blending are often looking for:

- A signature personal fragrance
- A well-rounded aroma that unfolds in stages (top, middle, base notes)
- A specific effect, such as a deeply calming bedtime blend or a mentally stimulating focus mix

We will examine the theory behind aroma families, how to structure a blend, and various ways to test and fine-tune your creations.

16.2 The Aroma Families

In perfumery and aromatherapy, experts often talk about aroma families. These group oils by their main scent profile:

1. **Citrus**: Lemon, orange, grapefruit, bergamot. Generally top notes that evaporate quickly.
2. **Floral**: Rose, jasmine, lavender, ylang ylang. Often middle notes that give softness or sweetness.
3. **Herbal**: Basil, clary sage, rosemary, marjoram. Can range from fresh to earthy. Often middle notes.
4. **Minty**: Peppermint, spearmint. Usually fresh and penetrating top notes.

5. **Earthy/Woody**: Cedarwood, patchouli, vetiver. Often base notes that last longer.
6. **Spicy**: Cinnamon, clove, black pepper, ginger. Can be warming, sometimes middle or base notes depending on the oil.
7. **Resinous**: Frankincense, myrrh. Often heavier base notes with a rich, balsamic aroma.

When you blend oils, you aim to combine these families in a way that either complements or contrasts them. For instance, a fresh citrus note might pair well with a woody base to create a balanced aroma that starts bright and ends warm.

16.3 Top, Middle, and Base Notes

In perfumery, oils are sometimes labeled as top, middle, or base notes based on how quickly they evaporate and how they shape the overall scent:

- **Top Notes**: Evaporate fast, create the first impression of a blend. Examples: lemon, bergamot, peppermint.
- **Middle Notes**: Form the heart of the blend, often last longer than top notes. Examples: lavender, rosemary, geranium.
- **Base Notes**: Evaporate slowly, linger as the final notes. Examples: patchouli, vetiver, sandalwood.

A common approach is to build blends with roughly 30% top notes, 50% middle notes, and 20% base notes. But this is not a strict rule—just a starting point. You might do 20-50-30, or another ratio, depending on personal preference or the purpose of the blend.

16.4 Creating a Structured Blend

Let us say you want to design a complex aroma. Here is a step-by-step method:

1. **Pick a Theme or Goal**

- Example: A calming, woodsy blend for evening relaxation.
2. **Select Potential Oils**
    - Base: Cedarwood, vetiver (woodsy, earthy).
    - Middle: Lavender, marjoram (relaxing, herbal).
    - Top: Bergamot or sweet orange (a gentle citrus uplift).
3. **Make Tiny Test Batches**
    - Use small amounts in a glass vial. For instance, start with a total of 10 drops so you can easily do percentages.
    - A sample ratio: 2 drops cedarwood, 1 drop vetiver, 4 drops lavender, 1 drop marjoram, 2 drops bergamot.
4. **Write Everything Down**
    - Keep track of exactly how many drops you used.
5. **Wait and Smell**
    - Smell right away, then again after 30 minutes, and again the next day. Some base notes bloom over time.
6. **Adjust**
    - If it is too woody, reduce vetiver. If it lacks brightness, add another drop of citrus.
7. **Test in Intended Application**
    - If it is for a diffuser, put a few drops in your diffuser with water. See if you like how it disperses.
    - If it is for a perfume, mix it in a carrier like jojoba and do a skin test.

16.5 Blending by Weight vs. Drops

Many hobbyists measure essential oils by drops. This is simple but not always precise, since drop size can vary by oil thickness and dropper type. Professionals sometimes use a small scale to measure in grams. This level of detail helps them repeat blends exactly.

- **Drops Method**: Easy for quick at-home experiments. Keep droppers consistent.
- **Scale Method**: More exact, good for larger batches or for turning a successful experiment into a product line.

If you do want to go deeper, you might invest in a small digital scale that can measure 0.01 grams. But for personal use, drops are usually enough if you do not mind slight variations.

16.6 Synergy and Accords

Synergy refers to the idea that when two or more oils mix, they can complement each other and create a result that is greater than the sum of their parts. For instance, mixing lavender and bergamot might smell better together than each one alone.

An **accord** is a blend of several oils that together form a unique "note" or sub-scent within a larger composition. For example, in perfumery, you might create a "rose accord" by mixing rose absolute, geranium, and palmarosa to achieve a rose-like effect without using pure rose (which can be expensive).

You can craft your own accords if you want to replicate certain scents or save on pricy oils.

16.7 Maturing and Letting Blends Rest

It is common for advanced blenders to let a mix rest for a few days or even weeks. Over time, molecules interact, sometimes changing the scent slightly. This process is akin to allowing a stew or sauce to develop deeper flavors overnight.

- **Short-Term Rest**: Even 24 hours can soften harsh edges.
- **Long-Term Rest**: For perfume blends, some people store them for 2–4 weeks before final evaluation.

During this resting period, keep the blend in a dark, cool place with a tight cap. Give it a gentle shake each day or so. After the chosen rest period, smell again and see if the blend has improved or changed.

16.8 Dilution for Different Purposes

- **Diffuser Blends**: Often you keep the oils undiluted in a small dropper bottle. You might add 4–6 drops of that synergy into your diffuser. This synergy bottle is your "master blend."
- **Topical Application**: If you are making a body oil, you need to mix your synergy into a carrier oil at the correct dilution (1–3% for general adult use, less for sensitive individuals).
- **Perfume**: Often requires an alcohol base (like perfumer's alcohol) or a carrier oil like jojoba. A typical concentration for a perfume oil might be 10–20% essential oils in the base, but it depends on how strong you want it and your skin sensitivity.

16.9 Rare Methods and Techniques

1. **Note Layering**: Create a small synergy of top notes, a synergy of middle notes, and a synergy of base notes separately. Then combine these smaller synergies. This can help you fine-tune each layer.
2. **Linear vs. Evolving Blends**: A linear blend smells similar from start to finish. An evolving blend changes over time, with top notes first, then a distinct heart, and finally the base.
3. **Using Headspace Technology**: Professionals sometimes capture the natural smell of a flower by analyzing the air around it (headspace) and then reconstruct that aroma with available oils or isolates. This is quite advanced and not typically done at home, but it is interesting to know.
4. **Blending According to Chemistry**: Some advanced folks consider chemical families (like monoterpenes, esters, aldehydes) to pair oils that share similar compounds or complement each other's properties. This can help produce stable blends or target specific goals (e.g., relaxing esters together).

16.10 Troubleshooting Blends

- **Too Sharp or Harsh**: Try adding a softening middle note (like a floral or a gentle herb). Sometimes a single drop of a base note like patchouli can ground a harsh blend.
- **Too Weak**: Increase the overall oil concentration, or add a stronger note. Some oils like black pepper or clove can boost the "presence" of a blend, but use them carefully.
- **Overly Sweet**: Mix in something fresh, minty, or slightly bitter (like a resinous or herbal note) to balance.
- **Unpleasant Dry-Down**: If the final lingering note on the skin is odd, check your base notes. They might need adjusting.

Keep detailed notes so you can fix issues in future versions. This record-keeping is key to becoming a skilled blender.

16.11 Example: Complex Relaxing Blend

Here is a hypothetical advanced blend aimed at deep relaxation:

- **Goal**: A slow-unfolding, comforting aroma that starts with a gentle brightness and settles into a soft, warm base.

Potential Oils

- Top (30%): 2 drops bergamot, 1 drop sweet orange
- Middle (50%): 4 drops lavender, 1 drop Roman chamomile
- Base (20%): 1 drop cedarwood, 1 drop vanilla oleoresin (if available)

Steps

1. In a small glass vial, place your base notes first: cedarwood, vanilla.
2. Add the middle notes: lavender, chamomile.
3. Add the top notes: bergamot, orange.
4. Swirl gently (do not shake too hard).

5. Let sit for an hour, then smell. If the citrus is not bright enough, add a drop more bergamot. If it is too sweet, add 1 drop of frankincense or perhaps a half-drop of clary sage.
6. Note the final count of each drop. Store and let it rest a day or two.

After resting, test it in a diffuser or as a 2% dilution in a carrier oil for a bath or massage. If it meets your goal of a comforting yet gently uplifting aroma, keep it. If not, do minor tweaks.

16.12 Making Signature Personal Perfumes

Some people love to create their own perfume to wear daily. This can be a statement of individuality. If you want to craft a personal signature:

1. **Pick Your Favorite Notes**
   - If you love florals, start with rose or jasmine. If you prefer fresh, maybe you pick a minty or citrus theme.
2. **Experiment in Vials**
   - Combine a floral middle with a warm base (like sandalwood or vanilla) and a light top (like bergamot).
   - You might end up with a ratio of 3:2:1 (middle:base:top) or something that pleases your nose.
3. **Move to an Alcohol Base**
   - Traditional perfumes are often in alcohol. You can buy perfume-grade alcohol or 90+% ethanol.
   - Mix the essential oil synergy in about 15–30% concentration, depending on how strong you want it.
4. **Age It**
   - Let the mixture sit for 2–4 weeks, shaking lightly every few days. This helps the scents meld.
5. **Test on Skin**
   - Your body chemistry can alter the fragrance. Check if you still love it after wearing it for a few hours.

16.13 Blending for Emotional or Physical Goals

Advanced aromatherapy blending is not just about smell. Some create blends to target certain wellness aims—like a "focus" blend or a "stress relief" synergy.

- **Focus Blend**: Might include rosemary (clarity), basil (alertness), lemon (uplifting).
- **Stress Relief**: Often uses lavender (calming), bergamot (mood-lifting), chamomile (soothing).
- **Easing Minor Discomfort**: Ginger, peppermint, and lavender are a popular trio in a massage oil for mild muscle tension.

Here, you combine your knowledge of aroma families with the known properties of each oil. Always stay within safe dilution levels.

16.14 Carrier Oils and Their Effect on Blends

Carrier oils themselves have scents (unless they are highly refined). For advanced projects, you might pick carriers that complement your essential oils:

1. **Jojoba**: Light, almost odorless. Good for most blends.
2. **Sweet Almond**: Mild, slightly nutty.
3. **Coconut (Fractionated)**: Mostly odorless, stays liquid.
4. **Rosehip**: Earthy, used for face serums, can alter the blend's scent slightly.
5. **Argan**: Nutty, can add a hint of aroma that might or might not fit your synergy.

If you want a pure representation of your essential oil synergy, pick an odorless carrier. If you do not mind a bit of extra earthy or nutty tone, use rosehip or argan.

16.15 Storing and Preserving Advanced Blends

- **Dark Glass Bottles**: Protect from sunlight.
- **Cool Environment**: Heat accelerates oxidation.
- **Label Clearly**: Write the date, formula (e.g., 2 drops lavender, 3 drops lemon, 1 drop cedarwood), and intended use.
- **Check Shelf Life**: Citrus oils can degrade faster than heavier oils like patchouli. A blend with lots of citrus might not last as long.

If you notice a sour or off smell, discard the blend.

16.16 Learning Through Trial and Error

Advanced blending is very much about practice. Be willing to make "mistakes" and toss out or rework attempts that do not turn out well. Over time, you will learn:

- Which oils go well together
- Which oils easily overpower others
- How to layer notes so the aroma changes smoothly over time
- How to fine-tune an aroma for your personal liking

Write notes in a blending journal. That way, when you hit upon a great combination, you can reproduce it.

16.17 Expanding Your Toolset

If you want to elevate your hobby:

1. **Aroma Strips** (Scent Strips): Paper strips dipped in a single oil or a test blend help you smell the fragrance without applying on skin. They are also called "fragrance blotters."
2. **Small Glass Vials**: For storing trial blends in small amounts.
3. **Perfumer's Alcohol**: Special alcohol that is odorless, letting your essential oils shine.

4. **A Notebook or Spreadsheet**: To record recipes, notes, modifications, and final thoughts.

16.18 Blending for Events or Seasonal Themes

You can tailor blends to certain times of year or special gatherings:

- **Winter Warmth**: Maybe a spicy blend with cinnamon, clove, and orange. Good for diffusing during cold months.
- **Spring Freshness**: Floral notes like lavender or geranium combined with a citrus top note.
- **Holiday Gatherings**: Pine, frankincense, and sweet orange to evoke a cozy environment.
- **Romantic Occasions**: Rose, ylang ylang, a hint of jasmine or vanilla for a soft, intimate feel.

This approach can create an aromatic atmosphere that matches the mood of the season or event.

16.19 Avoiding Common Pitfalls in Advanced Blending

- **Using Too Many Oils**: A blend with 10 different oils can become muddy or chaotic. Start with 2–4 oils. Only add more if needed.
- **Ignoring Personal Reactions**: Some people love patchouli, others cannot stand it. Always do a personal test.
- **Forgetting Evaporation Rates**: A top note might vanish in minutes, leaving you with mostly middle and base. Accept that top notes do not last long, or add a fixative base note (like sandalwood) to prolong them slightly.
- **Not Considering the Final Use**: A blend meant for a perfume might smell great in the bottle but differ on the skin. A diffuser blend might smell different once heated or dispersed.

16.20 Conclusion

Advanced blending is a creative process that merges art and a bit of science. It allows you to craft unique aromas for personal enjoyment, emotional support, or special occasions. By understanding aroma families, note placements, synergy, and proper ratios, you can go beyond simple two-oil mixes and develop richer, more refined scents.

Keep track of every step you take—both your successes and your failures—because each trial gives you insights into how oils interact. Over time, you will sharpen your nose and instincts, learning to predict how certain combinations will smell hours or even days later.

Whether you wish to form your own signature perfume, design a line of soothing roll-ons for friends, or simply enjoy the complexity of well-built scents around your home, advanced blending can be a fun skill. Combine curiosity, patience, and a love for fine aromas, and you will find that essential oils offer a nearly endless range of possibilities.

CHAPTER 17: Essential Oils in Massage and Physical Therapy

17.1 Introduction to Massage with Essential Oils

Massage is a practice that involves rubbing or pressing parts of the body to help relax muscles, improve circulation, and support ease of movement. It has been around for many centuries, appearing in the traditions of different cultures. Some people include essential oils in massages to add pleasant aromas and potential extra benefits for sore or tired muscles.

Physical therapy, on the other hand, often involves targeted exercises and methods to help people recover from injuries or manage chronic pain. Massage can be part of a larger physical therapy plan. In both cases, essential oils might serve as a gentle addition to improve comfort, mood, and relaxation.

This chapter will look at how to pick and use essential oils in massages or basic physical therapy routines, the safety guidelines you need to follow, and the ways in which certain oils might help. Remember that essential oils are not a replacement for expert care when facing serious health concerns, but they can be a small helper in a bigger plan.

17.2 Basic Principles of Massage

1. **Gentle Pressure**
    - In a typical massage, you apply pressure with your hands to the muscles. This pressure can vary from light stroking to deeper kneading, depending on the goal.
2. **Strokes and Movements**
    - Common massage movements include long gliding strokes, circular motions, tapping, or gentle shaking of muscles. Each method can help ease tension, improve blood flow, or calm the nervous system.
3. **Muscle Groups**

- Massages often target large muscle groups like those in the back, shoulders, legs, and neck. Some people may also target smaller areas like hands or feet.
4. **Relaxation and Breath**
    - During massage, the person usually breathes more slowly, which can add to the calm effect. Essential oils, with their soothing aromas, can add to this sense of ease.

A massage can be a short 5-10 minutes focusing on a specific area, or it can last an hour or more for a full-body approach. Essential oils can be blended into the massage oil or lotion for a pleasant scent and possible extra soothing effects.

17.3 Choosing the Right Oils for Massage

When adding essential oils to a massage routine, some people consider relaxing scents like lavender or chamomile. Others might prefer bright or warming scents like ginger or sweet marjoram for muscle support. Here are a few popular picks:

1. **Lavender (Lavandula angustifolia)**
    - Known for a gentle floral aroma.
    - Often linked with calming and easing mild tension.
    - Good for winding down after a busy day.
2. **Sweet Marjoram (Origanum majorana)**
    - Herbal, warm aroma.
    - Some people find it helps soothe tired or overworked muscles.
3. **Peppermint (Mentha x piperita)**
    - Cool, refreshing scent.
    - Can give a cooling feeling on the skin when diluted properly.
    - Useful for a pick-me-up effect, though it can be strong for some.
4. **Ginger (Zingiber officinale)**
    - Spicy, warm aroma.

- Some use it for improving the feel of stiff or tight muscles when blended with a carrier oil.
- Must be well-diluted to avoid skin irritation.
5. **Eucalyptus (Eucalyptus radiata)**
    - Fresh, clean scent often linked with a feeling of clear breathing.
    - Sometimes added to massage blends to refresh the body.
    - Keep amounts low if the person has sensitive skin or breathing concerns.
6. **Rosemary (Rosmarinus officinalis)**
    - Herbal, slightly sharp aroma.
    - Often linked to feelings of alertness.
    - Some people like it in sports massage blends for a stimulating effect.

When picking an oil, think about whether the person wants a calming vibe or a more energizing session. Also check that the chosen oil is safe for them, especially if they have allergies or sensitivities.

17.4 Dilution and Carrier Oils

Essential oils are strong. For massage, they must be diluted in a carrier oil or lotion before contact with skin. Common carrier oils include sweet almond, jojoba, fractionated coconut, or grapeseed oil. These are gentle on the skin and do not overshadow the aroma of the essential oils.

- **Typical Dilution**: About 1–3% essential oil is suitable for adult massage. That might be 1–3 drops of essential oil per teaspoon (5 mL) of carrier.
- **Sensitive or Elderly Skin**: Use an even lower dilution, around 0.5–1%.
- **Children**: Also around 0.25–1%, depending on age and expert advice.

Always do a patch test when using a new oil or blend to check for possible reactions. Put a little on the forearm, wait 24 hours, and see if there is any redness or itchiness.

17.5 Basic Massage Techniques

1. **Effleurage (Long Strokes)**
    - Light gliding movements with the whole hand.
    - Helps spread the oil, warms the muscles, and introduces touch.
2. **Petrissage (Kneading)**
    - Gentle pressing and rolling of the muscle.
    - Can help loosen tight spots and improve circulation.
3. **Friction**
    - Small, circular motions with fingertips or thumbs.
    - Targets deeper layers of muscle or connective tissue if done carefully.
4. **Tapotement (Tapping)**
    - Rhythmic tapping with the edges of the hands or fingertips.
    - Often used in sports massage to stimulate muscles.
5. **Vibration or Shaking**
    - Quick shaking of a limb or muscle group.
    - Can reduce tension and help the person relax.

You can mix these techniques in a session. The essential oil blend in the carrier oil helps your hands glide more smoothly and adds a pleasant aroma that might support relaxation or alertness.

17.6 Massage for Stress Relief

For people seeking calm, a simple routine might focus on the back, shoulders, or neck, where tension often builds. A typical process:

1. **Set the Mood**: Dim the lights, play quiet music, and diffuse a calming scent if desired.
2. **Warm the Oil**: Pour your carrier oil with the essential oil blend into your palms to warm it.
3. **Start with Light Strokes**: Use effleurage to spread the oil across the skin.

4. **Knead Tense Areas**: Gently press and release muscle knots around the shoulders or the base of the neck.
5. **Focus on Breathing**: Ask the person to take slow, steady breaths while you work on each area.
6. **Finish Lightly**: End with soft strokes. Let the person rest for a moment before getting up.

A blend example might be 2 drops lavender, 1 drop frankincense, and 1 drop sweet orange in 2 teaspoons of carrier oil.

17.7 Massage for Sports or Muscle Support

People who exercise or do physical work might use massage to help with post-workout soreness or to warm up muscles before an activity. Some might include a mild warming oil like ginger or black pepper (in a very small amount).

1. **Warm-Up**: Soft strokes to increase blood flow.
2. **Focus on Key Muscles**: Knead areas that feel stiff, such as calves, thighs, or back.
3. **Use Warming Oils**: A drop of ginger or black pepper in a tablespoon of carrier oil can add warmth, but always check for skin sensitivity.
4. **Avoid Over-Pressing**: Deep tissue work is best left to trained professionals if you are not certain of your technique.

If someone has a serious muscle injury or swelling, do not apply strong pressure. They may need rest, ice, or medical help first.

17.8 Essential Oils in Physical Therapy

In formal physical therapy, licensed professionals sometimes use oils as part of a broader set of methods, though not all clinics do. When they do, it might be for:

- **Relaxing Muscles Before Exercises**

- A short, gentle massage with essential oils to warm the tissues.
- **Improving Range of Motion**
  - If the client is more relaxed, they might move more freely in stretching or exercises.
- **Home Programs**
  - Therapists might suggest a mild massage oil for the patient to use at home, combined with their daily exercises.

Still, physical therapy focuses more on targeted exercises, manual movements, and other interventions (like ultrasound or electric stimulation). Essential oils are only a small addition if the therapist feels it helps. Always follow their guidance about which oils or methods to use if you are in a physical therapy program.

17.9 Special Cases: Joint Comfort and Mild Aches

Some individuals, especially older adults, might have mild aches in joints like knees or wrists. A gentle self-massage with a low-dilution essential oil blend could be soothing.

1. **Joint Circles**: Lightly rub around the joint in small circles, without pressing too hard on bones or tender areas.
2. **Warm Compress**: A warm towel (not too hot) placed on the joint after a light massage can further calm the area.
3. **Possible Oils**:
   - Ginger for a mild warming sensation.
   - Lavender or chamomile for calming.
   - Frankincense is sometimes used for older adults, though evidence is mixed on its effect.

Those with chronic conditions (like arthritis) should talk to a doctor or therapist before using essential oils. They might need a formal care plan, and some oils could be better avoided if there are medication interactions.

17.10 Creating Your Own Massage Blends

Making a blend for massage can be as simple as picking one or two essential oils. Or you can craft a more advanced synergy. Here is a simple process:

1. **Choose the Goal**: Relaxation, energizing, or muscle easing?
2. **Pick 2–3 Oils**: Maybe you want a floral note (like lavender), a herbal note (like rosemary), and a subtle base (like cedarwood).
3. **Decide on Dilution**: Usually 1–2% total essential oil in carrier. For example, for 2 tablespoons (30 mL) of carrier oil, 6–12 drops total of essential oil might be enough.
4. **Mix and Label**: Put them in a clean bottle. Label the name of the oils and date.
5. **Patch Test**: Check a small area on the skin. If no reaction, proceed.

When you find a blend that you love, store it in a dark glass container away from heat or sunlight. Use it within a few months, as carrier oils can go rancid over time.

17.11 Tips for a Good Massage Environment

- **Room Temperature**: The place should be warm so the person does not feel chilly when lying down.
- **Quiet Setting**: Loud noises can distract from relaxation. Soft background music or nature sounds are often used.
- **Clean Towels or Sheets**: Keep them ready to wipe off excess oil or to cover the person if they get cold.
- **Lighting**: Some people prefer low light or candlelight. Make sure there is enough visibility to perform the massage safely.
- **Scent Control**: If the essential oil is strong, air out the room afterward to avoid overwhelming others who might use the space.

17.12 Self-Massage Techniques

Not everyone can get a professional massage often. Self-massage is an option. You can apply oil to your hands or feet, or do simple neck or shoulder rubs. For example:

1. **Neck and Shoulders**:
   - Use your fingertips to press in circular motions, moving from the base of your neck outwards.
   - Keep your arms relaxed. If you feel too tense, shake out your arms, then continue.
2. **Feet**:
   - Sit in a comfortable chair, place one foot across your knee.
   - Apply a small amount of your chosen oil blend.
   - Rub the sole, moving from the heel to the toes. Use your thumb to apply gentle pressure.
3. **Hands and Wrists**:
   - Spread a little oil on the back of your hand and palm.
   - Use your other thumb to rub each finger, then the space between the fingers.
   - Circle around the wrist joint gently.
4. **Lower Back**:
   - Sometimes tricky to reach. You can use a tennis ball placed between your back and a wall, rolling gently to target muscles. A few drops of massage oil can be applied first if you can reach enough to rub it in.

Even a few minutes of self-massage can encourage relaxation or reduce mild stiffness. Be careful not to strain your arms if you have a large area to reach.

17.13 Cautions and When to Avoid Massage

- **Open Wounds or Rashes**: Do not massage over broken skin, rashes, or infections.
- **Inflammation or Swelling**: If an area is very hot or swollen, consult a medical professional.

- **Blood Clots**: People with known blood clots need medical advice before any deep tissue massage, as it may pose risks.
- **Unstable Health Conditions**: If someone has a heart problem or is at risk for complications, they should speak with a doctor first.
- **Sensitive Skin**: Use fewer essential oils or avoid them if the person has a history of strong skin reactions.

Always respect the body's signals. If the person feels pain or discomfort, ease off. If major symptoms arise, get professional help.

17.14 Rare Tips to Maximize the Experience

1. **Pre-Heat the Carrier Oil**: Placing the massage oil bottle in a bowl of warm water for a minute can create a cozy sensation when it touches the skin.
2. **Breathing Coordination**: Ask the person to inhale when you apply pressure and exhale when you release. This can deepen relaxation.
3. **Add a Warm Towel**: After finishing, lay a warm towel over the massaged area for a minute or two, helping the muscles stay relaxed.
4. **Set a Time Frame**: Even a 15-minute focused massage on the neck and shoulders can be effective. You do not need an hour if you are short on time.
5. **Blended Purposes**: Some people add small stretching exercises after a light massage to ease tight spots further.

17.15 Working with Professional Settings

If you are a massage therapist or physical therapist:

- **Speak with the Client**: Some might be allergic to certain oils. Others might not enjoy strong scents. Offer options or unscented alternatives.
- **Document**: Note which oils you used and the client's response. This helps create a consistent experience if they return.

- **Follow Regulations**: Some areas have rules about which methods are allowed in therapy settings. Ensure you comply with local guidelines.
- **Educate Clients**: Show them simple home techniques if they wish to continue mild self-care between sessions.

For individuals receiving therapy, always tell your therapist about any allergies or special conditions. They can adjust the approach accordingly.

17.16 Combining Massage with Other Modalities

- **Warm Baths**: A short bath with essential oils (properly diluted) before a massage can soften muscles and make the session smoother.
- **Aromatherapy Diffusion**: You can also diffuse a calming oil in the room while massaging.
- **Heat or Ice**: Some injuries respond better to gentle heat or cold packs, so check with a doctor or therapist if you need those instead of direct massage.
- **Gentle Exercise**: Light stretching or yoga after massage might maintain flexibility.

17.17 Sample Massage Blend Recipes

1. **Relaxing Lavender Blend**
    - 2 tablespoons sweet almond oil (about 30 mL)
    - 6 drops lavender essential oil
    - 2 drops cedarwood essential oil
    - Good for bedtime or a calm evening session.
2. **Warming Ginger Blend**
    - 1 tablespoon jojoba oil (15 mL)
    - 1 drop ginger essential oil
    - 2 drops sweet marjoram essential oil
    - 1 drop orange essential oil

- Apply to stiff muscles gently. Test on a small area first, as ginger can be spicy.
3. **Energizing Peppermint Blend**
    - 2 tablespoons fractionated coconut oil
    - 3 drops peppermint essential oil
    - 3 drops rosemary essential oil
    - This can feel refreshing, especially for a midday pick-me-up. Avoid eyes and face area, as peppermint can be quite strong.

17.18 Massage for Office or Desk Workers

Many people who work at desks develop stiffness in the neck, shoulders, and lower back. A quick self-massage at the desk, using a small roller bottle of a mild essential oil blend, can help:

1. **Neck Roll-On**:
    - 10 mL roller bottle, fill with fractionated coconut oil.
    - Add 2 drops lavender and 1 drop peppermint.
    - Shake and roll on the back of the neck, then rub gently.
2. **Shoulder Tension**:
    - Place a tennis ball behind your back against a wall.
    - Roll up and down to apply pressure to stiff spots in the shoulders.
    - If you like, apply a small dab of massage oil first so the ball can move smoothly.
3. **Short Breaks**:
    - Even 2-3 minutes every hour can reduce stress buildup. Combine with posture checks and gentle stretching.

17.19 Improving Physical Therapy Homework

If your doctor or therapist gave you exercises to do at home, a short warm-up with essential oils can make them more comfortable:

- **Self-Massage**: Rub tight muscles lightly for a minute or two.
- **Gentle Joint Circles**: Move the joint slowly within a pain-free range.
- **Proceed with Exercises**: Follow your therapist's instructions for sets and reps.
- **Cool Down**: End with another quick rub or a soothing foot soak if needed.

This approach can keep you consistent in your therapy plan and may make the exercises feel more pleasant. But always follow the advice of your healthcare provider regarding best methods for your condition.

17.20 Conclusion

Massage and physical therapy are about supporting the body's comfort, movement, and relaxation. Essential oils can be a friendly addition, providing pleasing scents and a smoother glide for the hands during massage. Choices like lavender, sweet marjoram, or peppermint can match different needs—be it calming, warming, or refreshing. Proper dilution, safe handling, and simple techniques go a long way in making the experience beneficial.

Whether you are a professional or simply looking after your own well-being at home, a thoughtful blend of essential oils can turn an ordinary massage into a gentle, enjoyable session. Focus on the basics: the right oil, safe dilution, good technique, and clear communication about comfort and allergies. Used wisely, essential oils can make each massage session more pleasant, be it for easing stress, supporting muscle recovery, or adding a soothing scent to a physical therapy plan.

CHAPTER 18: Essential Oils in Pet Care

18.1 Introduction to Using Essential Oils for Pets

Many people consider pets as part of the family, and they want to use natural methods to keep them comfortable or smelling pleasant. Some might think about applying essential oils or diffusing them in the home to help with pet odor or minor issues like pests. However, animals have different bodies than humans, and some essential oils can be harmful to them.

This chapter will explore how certain essential oils can be used around pets, plus the strong guidelines you must follow. We will focus mainly on cats and dogs, as they are common household pets. We will also mention birds and other small animals briefly. Always note that a vet's advice should come first, especially if your pet has health conditions.

18.2 Why Pets Respond Differently

1. **Differences in Metabolism**
   - Animals, especially cats, lack certain liver enzymes that help break down chemicals found in essential oils. This can make them more sensitive or lead to toxicity if used incorrectly.
2. **Sensitivity to Smells**
   - Dogs have a strong sense of smell, often much sharper than humans. A scent that seems mild to you can be overwhelming to them.
   - Cats can also be very reactive to strong fragrances.
3. **Self-Grooming**
   - Many animals, like cats and dogs, lick their fur. If an essential oil is on their coat, they might ingest it. That can lead to digestive troubles or worse.
4. **Weight and Body Size**
   - Pets, especially small ones, weigh much less than humans. A tiny amount of essential oil that is mild for us can be a big dose for them.

Because of these factors, using essential oils near pets requires caution and often a discussion with a vet who understands essential oils.

18.3 Oils to Avoid with Pets

Some oils are widely considered risky or harmful around cats and dogs. This list is not complete, but it includes several known problem oils:

- **Tea Tree (Melaleuca alternifolia)**: While popular for humans, it can be toxic to pets if ingested or applied in strong amounts.
- **Wintergreen (Gaultheria procumbens)**: Contains methyl salicylate, which can be dangerous to pets.
- **Pine (Pinus species)**: Can irritate their respiratory system or skin if used incorrectly.
- **Cinnamon (Cinnamomum zeylanicum)**: Often too hot and can cause mouth or skin irritation if pets come into contact.
- **Citrus Oils (Lemon, Orange, Bergamot, etc.)**: Some cats are very sensitive to these. They may cause drooling, wobbliness, or more severe issues if ingested.
- **Eucalyptus (Eucalyptus globulus)**: Can be irritating to some animals, especially if they have respiratory conditions.

If you see a product labeled for pets that contains such oils, be sure it is in a safe form and very low concentration under veterinary guidance. But in general, it is wise to keep these oils away from animals unless you have expert advice.

18.4 Safe Practices for Diffusing Around Pets

1. **Ventilation**
    - Always run a diffuser in a well-ventilated area. Keep a window or door open so your pet can leave if the scent bothers them.
2. **Short Durations**

- Limit diffusion to 15–30 minutes at a time. Do not run it constantly.
- Watch your pet's behavior. If they sneeze, hide, or seem uneasy, turn off the diffuser and air out the room.

3. **Choose Mild Oils**
   - If you must diffuse, pick oils that are considered gentler, like a tiny amount of lavender.
   - Still, keep in mind some animals might not tolerate even those.
4. **Location**
   - Place the diffuser high on a shelf where the pet cannot knock it over or inhale the mist directly.
5. **Monitor Signs**
   - If the pet coughs, wheezes, drools, trembles, or acts oddly, turn off the diffuser and call a vet.

Many experts suggest avoiding routine essential oil diffusion in the same room as pets, especially if the oils are strong or the pet cannot leave the space.

18.5 Using Essential Oils Topically on Pets

Some pet owners want to apply a diluted oil to the pet's fur for odor control or mild skin issues. This must be done very carefully:

1. **Vet Approval**
   - Always ask your veterinarian first. They might suggest a safer product or say to skip essential oils altogether.
2. **Proper Dilution**
   - For dogs, a common suggestion is a very low amount, like 0.5% or less. For cats, many vets say avoid topical essential oils entirely.
3. **Avoid Face and Paws**
   - Pets lick their paws and face. They might ingest the oil if it is put there.
   - Also avoid eyes, nose, mouth, or ears.
4. **Patch Test**

- Try a small spot on the back (where the pet cannot easily lick). Wait 24 hours. If there is no redness or irritation, it may be okay to apply gently.
5. **Observe**
    - If the pet starts grooming intensely, drooling, or showing confusion, wash off the oil with mild soap and water and contact a vet if symptoms persist.

Remember, cats in particular are known to be very sensitive. Many experts strongly advise against direct application of essential oils on felines unless a vet with specialized knowledge has recommended it.

18.6 Common Pet-Related Uses People Attempt

1. **Flea or Tick Control**
    - Some owners try essential oils to repel fleas or ticks. But oils like citronella, cedarwood, or lemongrass can still be harmful if used incorrectly, especially for cats.
    - Some vet-approved natural products contain these oils in very low concentrations. Always double-check.
2. **Calming Anxiety**
    - A few individuals diffuse lavender or chamomile to help a nervous dog during storms. But again, the dog should be able to leave the room if they dislike the smell.
    - Some dogs may benefit from specially formulated dog-safe calming sprays.
3. **Odor Control**
    - People sometimes want to get rid of "dog smell" or litter box odors. They might diffuse oils or spray an essential oil mix. This can irritate the pet's nose.
    - Instead, use natural ventilation or pet-safe deodorizers recommended by vets.
4. **Minor Skin Irritations**
    - Some try diluted chamomile or lavender on a dog's minor hot spot. But best to ask a vet to confirm that it is safe.

While these uses are common, each comes with possible risks for your pet's health. Weigh the pros and cons carefully.

18.7 Signs of Essential Oil Toxicity in Pets

If a pet is exposed to an unsafe oil or too much oil, signs may include:

- **Drooling or Foaming** at the mouth
- **Vomiting** or diarrhea
- **Shaking, Tremors, or Seizures**
- **Trouble Walking** (staggering, loss of balance)
- **Breathing Difficulty** or panting
- **Weakness or Lethargy**
- **Skin Irritation** or redness where the oil was applied
- **Behavior Changes** like hiding, restlessness, or vocalizing

If you see any of these, remove your pet from the area and contact a vet right away. If oil is on the fur, wash gently with mild soap and rinse thoroughly.

18.8 Bird and Small Animal Concerns

Birds have very sensitive respiratory systems. Strong odors, smoke, or fumes can harm them quickly. Small animals like hamsters, rabbits, or guinea pigs can also be sensitive. In general:

- **Do Not Diffuse** strong oils in a room with caged birds or small pets.
- **Ensure Proper Ventilation** or move them to another room if you do choose to diffuse.
- **Never Apply Oils** directly to the fur or feathers of small pets.

Due to their delicate systems, many vets advise against using essential oils around birds altogether.

18.9 Alternatives to Essential Oils for Pet Care

If you are unsure, there are other natural or less risky options:

1. **Proper Grooming**
    - Regular baths (with vet-approved shampoo), brushing, and nail trimming help keep a pet clean and healthy.
2. **Good Hygiene**
    - Clean bedding and litter boxes often to reduce smells.
    - Wash your pet's blankets or toys with mild, pet-safe detergents.
3. **Vet-Recommended Flea or Tick Products**
    - Many effective products exist that are tested for safety.
    - Natural brands might have lower amounts of certain extracts, but they still need proper oversight to ensure they work and are safe.
4. **Calming Products**
    - Special pheromone diffusers (like synthetic dog-appeasing pheromone) can help anxious pets without the potential hazards of essential oils.
5. **Good Ventilation**
    - Simply opening windows or using fans can help with odors, avoiding the need for strong fragrances.

18.10 Rare Tips for Limited, Safer Use

If, after talking to a vet, you still plan to use essential oils:

1. **Short Trials**
    - Start with 5–10 minutes of mild diffusion in a large room while the pet has free access to leave. Observe the pet's behavior carefully.
2. **Pick One Oil**
    - Do not blend multiple oils. This keeps it simpler to spot problems.
    - Lavender is often considered one of the least problematic for some dogs, but that is not guaranteed safe.
3. **Use a Personal Inhaler**
    - Instead of diffusing in the entire space, consider a personal inhaler for yourself if you want to enjoy the scent. That way, you do not fill the room with the aroma.

4. **Store Oils Securely**
    - Keep essential oil bottles where pets cannot knock them over or chew them.
    - Animals might be drawn to the smell or the shape of the bottle.
5. **Never Force It**
    - If your pet shows any sign of discomfort, remove the source.

18.11 Creating a Pet-Safe Environment at Home

- **Pet Zones**: Keep an oil-free zone where your pet spends most of their time, such as a living room corner or a bed area.
- **Designated Aromatherapy Time**: If you enjoy a diffuser, use it in a separate room with the door closed. Ventilate afterward before letting your pet inside.
- **Watch the Floor**: If oil drips on the floor, clean it up so the pet does not lick it or get it on their paws.

18.12 Pet-Safe Cleaning

Many people who love essential oils also like natural cleaning. But if you have pets, pick your cleaning methods carefully:

1. **Avoid Strong Oils in Floor Cleaners**
    - Pets walk on floors and may lick their paws later.
2. **Rinse Thoroughly**
    - Whether cleaning bowls, cages, or litter boxes, rinse well to remove any residue.
3. **Mild Vinegar Solutions**
    - Often safer for surfaces pets touch.
4. **Read Labels**
    - Some "natural" cleaners might still have oils that are risky for animals.

18.13 Dealing with Pet Anxiety or Stress

If your goal is to help a stressed dog or cat:

- **Try Behavior Training**: Work with a trainer or behaviorist to address the root cause of anxiety.
- **Pheromone Products**: As mentioned, these mimic natural cues that can calm some pets.
- **Safe Spaces**: Provide a quiet, comfy area where the pet feels secure.
- **Consult a Vet**: In some cases, medication or special diets help with severe anxiety.

Essential oils may not be the best solution, and for some pets, they could even add stress if the scent is too strong.

18.14 Real-Life Cases: Successes and Risks

- **Success Story**: A dog owner used a single drop of diluted lavender on a bandanna near the dog's neck (not on the skin) during thunderstorms. The dog seemed calmer. The key was that the dog could remove themselves from the scent if bothered. This was done under a vet's guidance.
- **Risk Story**: A cat owner diffused tea tree oil to freshen the living room. The cat developed drooling and weakness. A vet found signs of toxicity, and the cat needed urgent care. The cat recovered, but it served as a warning about the dangers of certain oils.

Each pet reacts differently. What worked for one may not be safe for another. This is why a cautious approach and individual guidance are so important.

18.15 Approaches for Groomers and Pet Spas

Some professional pet groomers or spas use mild essential oil sprays or shampoos. If you run or visit a grooming service:

- **Check Formulations**: Ensure the product is specifically designed and tested for pets.
- **Low Concentration**: The final product should have a tiny amount of essential oil, if any.
- **Allow Pet Owners to Opt Out**: Some might not want any essential oils near their pet.
- **Watch for Reactions**: If a dog or cat shows discomfort, rinse them well and switch to unscented products.

18.16 Bird Owners: Extra Caution

Since birds are so sensitive:

1. **No Direct Use**: Do not apply oils to feathers or feet.
2. **Avoid Diffusion**: Even mild oils can harm a bird's respiratory system.
3. **Clean Air**: Keep the cage in a well-ventilated area, free from strong scents.

If you suspect your bird has inhaled something harmful, move them to fresh air and contact a vet.

18.17 Less Common Pets: Reptiles, Rodents, and Others

Reptiles, like snakes or lizards, have their own sensitivity to chemicals. Rodents (like guinea pigs or hamsters) are small and fragile. The general rule is the same: do not experiment with essential oils on or around them unless a vet with exotic pet knowledge says it is okay.

18.18 Signs You Should Stop Using Essential Oils with Pets

- **Behavior Changes**: Hiding, aggression, or refusal to enter a room that smells like oils.
- **Respiratory Issues**: Rapid breathing, wheezing, or coughing.
- **Skin Problems**: Rash, dryness, or itching in areas where the pet might contact oil.
- **Neurological Symptoms**: Tremors, stumbling, confusion.
- **Digestive Problems**: Vomiting, diarrhea after exposure.

Stopping early can prevent serious harm. Clean the area, wash the pet if there is direct contact, and call the vet if symptoms seem serious.

18.19 If You Really Want a Light Scent

Some pet owners just want their dog or cat to smell a bit fresher. In that case:

1. **Pet-Safe Cologne or Sprays**: Certain pet product brands make mild, tested fragrances.
2. **DIY Light Herb Sprays**: A weak herbal tea (like chamomile or rosemary tea) cooled and lightly misted can add a pleasant smell without the concentration of an essential oil. Test it on a small area first.
3. **Frequent Bathing** (for dogs): Use a mild, pet-friendly shampoo. For cats, bathing is less common, but some cats tolerate it.
4. **Healthy Diet**: Sometimes a strong odor can come from poor diet or dental issues, so address root causes.

18.20 Conclusion

Essential oils can be appealing for natural pet care, but in reality, they often pose more risks than benefits. Cats, birds, small rodents, and even many dogs are much more sensitive to these powerful plant extracts than humans. If you do decide to use essential oils around your pet, always do so with serious caution and, ideally, with a vet's guidance.

Many safer alternatives exist for dealing with pet odors, fleas, or minor skin troubles. Good grooming habits, vet-approved products, and a clean living space might be all you need. If you truly wish to introduce essential oils, keep the concentration extremely low, allow the pet to leave the area, and watch for any signs of discomfort or toxicity. When in doubt, skip the oils. Your pet's health and comfort come first.

Used carefully—or, in many cases, avoided—essential oils can fit into a pet-friendly home. But remember that "natural" does not always mean "safe," especially when it comes to animals with unique biology. Stay informed, talk with a knowledgeable vet, and focus on methods that keep your furry or feathered friends safe and content.

CHAPTER 19: Setting Up an Essential Oil Business

19.1 Introduction to the Essential Oil Industry

Starting a business in the essential oil field can be both exciting and complex. You might want to sell individual oils, create custom blends, or offer related products like skincare or household items. This chapter will outline some key steps to consider when planning an essential oil enterprise, from sourcing raw materials to final marketing. While no single path suits everyone, you can adapt these guidelines to your situation.

The global demand for essential oils is significant. People use them for relaxation, household cleaning, skincare, or personal fragrance. However, the market is also crowded, and competition can be tough. To stand out, you need a clear strategy, good quality standards, and an honest message about what your products can offer.

19.2 Deciding on a Business Model

Before diving into the details, think about what kind of essential oil business you want. Some common models:

1. **Retailing Single Oils**
    - You might import or buy oils wholesale, then repackage them under your brand.
    - This can be simpler if you find a reliable supplier, but you must ensure purity and consistency.
2. **Creating Blends or Specialty Products**
    - You develop your own recipes, such as diffuser blends, massage oils, bath soaks, or skincare items.
    - This requires knowledge of blending, product formulation, and local regulations for cosmetics or body care.
3. **Private Labeling**

- A manufacturer produces oils or blends, and you add your own label.
- You focus on branding, marketing, and distribution, leaving production to a third party.

4. **Direct Selling or Network Marketing**
    - Some companies run a multi-level approach, where sellers join and promote products.
    - This can involve recruiting a sales force. It's a special model with its own rules and image.
5. **Educational Services**
    - You might sell a small product line, but focus on workshops, consulting, or aromatherapy courses.
    - This requires recognized credentials in aromatherapy or a related area.

Clarify which path suits your skills and resources. Each approach has different demands on inventory, capital, and marketing style.

19.3 Market Research and Target Audience

Understanding your potential buyers is vital:

1. **Demographics**
    - Are you aiming for wellness enthusiasts? Spa owners? Busy parents? Corporate offices looking for natural solutions?
2. **Customer Preferences**
    - Some customers want pure single oils; others want ready-to-use blends.
    - Look at trends like aromatherapy for stress relief, natural cleaning, or green cosmetics.
3. **Competitor Analysis**
    - Find out what similar businesses offer. Check their product lines, pricing, packaging, and marketing angles.
    - Identify gaps—maybe none focus on child-safe blends or seniors, or perhaps there's a shortage of budget-friendly oils in your region.
4. **Price Range**

- Many essential oils can be pricey. Figure out if your audience wants premium or mid-range products.
- If you're targeting the high-end market, your branding and packaging must reflect that.

Gathering market data helps you tailor your brand. This might involve online surveys, local focus groups, or speaking with potential customers at markets or fairs. Real feedback can guide product decisions.

19.4 Legal Requirements and Certifications

Regulations for essential oils vary depending on where you live. Some countries classify them as cosmetics if used on the body, or as food flavorings if used for cooking. Key points to check:

1. **Business Registration**
   - Obtain a business license, register your brand name, and follow local tax rules.
2. **Labeling Laws**
   - You might need to list botanical names, possible allergens, safe usage instructions, or disclaimers.
   - Overblown health claims can attract legal trouble.
3. **Import/Export Rules**
   - If you buy oils from overseas or plan to ship products internationally, follow customs and safety regulations.
   - Some plant materials are restricted to protect against invasive species or environmental harm.
4. **Certification**
   - You may want to seek organic certification if your oils come from farms that do not use certain pesticides.
   - Fair trade or sustainable harvest certifications can appeal to eco-conscious buyers.
   - These processes take time and money, so plan carefully.

Consult legal and regulatory experts, especially if you blend oils for personal care items. Each region has different standards for cosmetics, labeling, and product safety testing.

19.5 Finding Reliable Suppliers

Securing high-quality oils is the heart of your business. If your oils are impure or mislabeled, your brand's reputation can suffer. Steps to pick good suppliers:

1. **Look for Transparency**
    - Reliable suppliers share information about distillation methods, plant origins, and any testing they do (like GC-MS reports).
2. **Test Samples**
    - Order small samples from potential suppliers. Evaluate scent, clarity, color, and packaging.
    - If possible, pay for a third-party lab test on random samples to confirm purity.
3. **Check Farming and Harvesting Practices**
    - Ask how the plants are grown and harvested. Overharvesting certain species can be unsustainable.
    - If an oil is endangered or in short supply (like sandalwood from some regions), this can pose ethical or environmental concerns.
4. **Consistency**
    - Plant yields can vary from year to year. Make sure the supplier can provide a stable supply of your most important oils.
    - You might diversify, working with multiple suppliers to avoid disruptions if one fails.
5. **Pricing and MOQ (Minimum Order Quantity)**
    - Suppliers often have bulk requirements. Make sure you can handle the order size and storage.
    - Extremely cheap oils might be adulterated, so compare prices across a few sources.

19.6 Branding and Packaging

To stand out in a crowded market, invest in thoughtful branding:

1. **Brand Identity**
    - Decide on the vibe: Are you rustic and homemade? Sleek and modern? Science-oriented?
    - Pick colors, fonts, and a logo that convey your theme.
2. **Storytelling**
    - Consumers like to know the background: Where do the oils come from? Who are the farmers or distillers?
    - Share your personal reason for loving essential oils, or your mission to provide pure, honest products.
3. **Label Design**
    - Include oil name, botanical name, origin, and recommended uses or cautions.
    - Keep it readable. Some countries require a specific format for ingredient lists.
4. **Bottling Choices**
    - Usually, essential oils come in amber or cobalt glass bottles to protect from light.
    - For blends, you might use roller bottles or droppers.
    - Consider child-resistant caps if required by law.

In an online marketplace, a clean, professional look can build trust. Product photography should highlight the bottle design and, if relevant, the source plants or appealing backgrounds.

19.7 Pricing Your Products

Finding the right price means balancing costs and customer willingness to pay. Factors to include:

1. **Cost of Goods**
    - The actual cost of oil, bottles, labels, shipping, storage, plus any added carrier oils or ingredients.
2. **Overheads**
    - Rent (if you have a workspace), insurance, licenses, staff salaries, marketing, website fees, and more.
3. **Profit Margin**

- You need a margin to cover your time and ensure the business can grow or handle unexpected costs.
4. **Market Position**
    - If you aim for premium status, your price might be higher than mainstream options. The brand story and packaging should match that.
    - A budget-friendly approach requires higher volume sales to stay profitable.

Look at competitor prices. If your oils are more expensive, show why they're better—maybe they're organic, fair trade, or come from specialty farms. If you go cheaper, ensure you still provide decent quality.

19.8 Distribution Channels

Think about where and how you will sell:

1. **Online Store**
    - Platforms like Shopify or Etsy let you reach a wide audience quickly.
    - You handle order packing, shipping, and customer service.
    - SEO (Search Engine Optimization) and social media presence are key.
2. **Local Shops and Spas**
    - Approach gift stores, wellness centers, or salons. Show them samples, wholesale pricing, and marketing materials.
    - A smaller supply chain can be simpler, but the buyer might want a cut of the retail price.
3. **Markets and Events**
    - Farmers' markets or craft fairs let you connect with customers face-to-face.
    - You can offer sniff tests or mini demos.
4. **Direct Sales**
    - Some entrepreneurs hold home parties or small workshops. This can be personal but takes time and planning.
5. **Wholesale to Other Brands**
    - If you produce large quantities, you can be a supplier to smaller businesses or re-branding companies.

- Price your wholesale products carefully so you still make a profit.

Each channel has pros and cons. If you start small, you can test local events or an online store. Over time, expand into bigger channels if you have the stock and marketing budget.

19.9 Marketing and Promotion

A strong marketing plan can help you stand out:

1. **Website and Social Media**
   - Post product photos, usage tips, and behind-the-scenes glimpses of how you source or blend oils.
   - Platforms like Instagram, Pinterest, or Facebook can be effective for visuals and short educational posts.
2. **Educational Content**
   - Blog articles or short videos showing how to safely use a blend in a diffuser, or how to make a simple DIY cleaner.
   - This positions you as a knowledgeable resource, not just a seller.
3. **Email Newsletters**
   - Gather customer emails at markets or through your site.
   - Send updates on new blends, seasonal promotions, or special bundles.
4. **Influencer or Affiliate Partnerships**
   - Aromatherapists, wellness coaches, or natural-living influencers might highlight your products.
   - Offer them a sample or affiliate code. If their followers trust them, you can reach more buyers.
5. **Customer Reviews and Testimonials**
   - Encourage happy customers to leave honest feedback on your site or social media pages.
   - Respond politely to negative feedback, focusing on solutions.

Staying genuine is key. Avoid unrealistic health promises. Instead, share safe usage tips and your brand's unique approach to quality.

19.10 Setting Up Production and Storage

If you blend oils, you need a clean, organized space:

1. **Workspace Basics**
    - A separate area to keep tools, bottles, droppers, and oils.
    - Surfaces that are easy to wipe down if spills happen.
2. **Proper Ventilation**
    - Some oils release strong fumes. A well-ventilated room or fan can help.
    - Keep flammable oils away from heat sources.
3. **Labeling Station**
    - Have a system so each product is labeled correctly with batch numbers, best-before dates, and more.
4. **Storage**
    - Essential oils often stay stable longer in cool, dark places.
    - Large containers or drums might need temperature control.
    - Keep an inventory system so you know which oils are nearing expiration.
5. **Quality Control**
    - Keep track of each batch. If you notice a difference in scent or color, retest before selling.
    - If an oil is oxidized or smells off, do not sell it.

19.11 Scaling Up the Business

As sales grow, challenges appear:

1. **Managing Inventory**
    - You might need more space or staff to handle packing and shipping.
    - If you run out of a popular oil, you risk losing customers to competitors.
2. **Automation**
    - Online platforms can automate shipping labels or track orders.
    - Email marketing tools can handle promotional campaigns.

3. **Hiring Help**
    - You could hire someone for packing, customer service, or social media.
    - Train them on product details so they can answer questions accurately.
4. **Cash Flow**
    - Large orders for bottles or raw oils can be expensive.
    - Plan your finances so you do not overbuy or underbuy.
    - Keep a buffer for unexpected costs, like shipping delays or price spikes in raw materials.

19.12 Building Trust and Credibility

The essential oil market faces many claims about purity and results. Customers can be wary:

1. **Third-Party Testing**
    - Sharing GC-MS reports or certifications shows you are transparent.
    - This can justify premium pricing if the test proves high purity.
2. **Educational Approach**
    - Outline realistic benefits and safe usage.
    - Avoid hype words that promise cures or extreme results.
3. **Consistent Quality**
    - If customers love a specific lavender batch, make sure the next batch is close in aroma and strength.
    - Sudden changes can create doubt.
4. **Responsive Customer Service**
    - Handle complaints or inquiries quickly and politely.
    - Offer replacements or refunds when appropriate to maintain goodwill.

19.13 Handling Challenges and Liability

When dealing with items that can be applied to skin or used in the home, consider:

1. **Allergic Reactions**
   - Advise patch tests. Label your products with disclaimers.
   - Make no claims that it's 100% risk-free for every person.
2. **Safety Warnings**
   - Mention phototoxic oils or those not recommended for pregnant individuals or pets.
   - Even if disclaimers reduce sales, it helps keep your brand honest and safe.
3. **Insurance**
   - Product liability insurance can protect you if someone misuses the oil or has an adverse reaction.
   - Check if your policy covers international orders if you ship abroad.
4. **Competition and Pricing Pressures**
   - Over time, new sellers might show up with lower prices. Continue to emphasize quality, sustainability, and good service.

19.14 Exploring Secondary Products

Once you have a foothold, you can expand:

1. **Cosmetics and Skincare**
   - If local laws permit, create creams, lotions, or bath bombs with your oils.
   - This requires additional testing for shelf stability.
2. **Candles or Wax Melts**
   - Many essential oil brands add candles to their line. Natural wax (like soy or beeswax) plus pure oils can be a big draw.
   - Scent throw testing is important here (how well the aroma disperses when burned).
3. **Gift Sets**

- Bundles for birthdays, holidays, or corporate gifts.
- Combine a few oils or blends in a nice box, possibly with diffusers or small educational booklets.

4. **Workshops or Classes**
    - Teach basic blending or usage classes online or in-person.
    - Participants might buy oils on the spot if you have them ready for sale.

Balancing multiple product lines can be complex, so expand gradually and keep quality at the forefront.

19.15 Success Stories and Failures

Examples (without naming specific brands):

- **Small Town Boutique**: A person started selling homemade lavender body oil at a local farmer's market. They focused on one item at first. Over time, customers began asking for more scents, so they introduced more blends. Now they run a small storefront and do steady business online.
- **Overextension**: Another seller launched a website with over 50 different essential oils, plus skincare and candles, all at once. They struggled with inventory, lost track of batch dates, and had a series of out-of-stock items. Customers got frustrated, and the brand's reputation suffered.

It pays to start small and grow in stages. Master your supply chain and keep your brand message clear.

19.16 Rare Tips for Growth

- **Limited Edition Releases**: Occasionally offer a specialty blend with rare oils. This can generate interest.
- **Partner with Local Farmers**: If you have local farms growing lavender or rosemary, create a "farm-to-bottle" storyline.

- **Cross-Promotion**: Work with yoga studios, wellness coaches, or restaurants that use essential oils in cooking. You might host joint events or put out sample kits in their waiting area.
- **Subscription Boxes**: Offer monthly or quarterly boxes with curated oils or blends for different themes (like winter wellness, spring cleaning, etc.).

19.17 Monitoring Trends

Stay aware of shifts in consumer behavior:

- **Eco-Friendly Packaging**: People increasingly prefer less plastic, more sustainable materials.
- **Sustainable Sourcing**: Overharvesting can hurt plant populations. Some customers want to see that your brand cares for the environment.
- **Science and Research**: More consumers read about actual studies on essential oils. They want data, not just anecdotes.
- **Global or Cultural Influences**: New floral oils from different regions might become popular. Seasonal fads may impact your short-term blends.

Adapting to these trends thoughtfully can keep your brand relevant.

19.18 Time Management and Self-Care

Running an essential oil business can be demanding. You need to handle orders, talk to customers, manage finances, and maybe create new products. A few pointers:

1. **Set Work Hours**
    - If you run this from home, keep boundaries so you do not work 24/7.
2. **Delegate**
    - Outsource tasks like bookkeeping if that frees you to focus on product quality or marketing.

3. **Avoid Burnout**
    - Use your own products to relax—a short aromatherapy break might remind you why you started this venture.
4. **Stay Organized**
    - Simple project management tools or spreadsheets can track tasks, deadlines, and ideas.

19.19 Building a Long-Term Vision

A business plan goes beyond immediate sales. Aim for a stable, ethical brand that can last:

- **Continual Product Improvement**: Gather feedback. Maybe rework a blend if customers say it's too strong or lacks depth.
- **Community Involvement**: Sponsor local events or charities that align with natural living or environmental care.
- **Future Partnerships**: Could you partner with hotels for signature room fragrances? Or create a line for a major spa chain? Dream big but plan carefully.
- **Exit Strategy**: Some owners eventually sell their brand or hand it to family. Keep good records in case you want that option.

19.20 Conclusion

Starting an essential oil business combines creativity with a strong sense of responsibility. Sourcing top-notch materials, understanding the market, building trust, and managing legal or labeling rules can be complex. Yet, with thoughtful planning, clear brand identity, and consistent quality control, you can carve out a space in the market.

Keep learning about new oils, blending methods, and changing consumer tastes. Maintain open communication with your customers, treat them fairly, and be transparent about what you offer. Over time, a well-run essential oil venture can provide a steady income, personal fulfillment, and a way to share your passion for the natural aromas that drew you into this field in the first place.

CHAPTER 20: Future Trends and Ongoing Research

20.1 Introduction to Emerging Directions

Essential oils have a long history, but they keep evolving with modern science, technology, and consumer demands. Researchers around the world continue to study their chemical makeup, potential uses, and safety aspects. At the same time, new consumer trends appear—like advanced diffusers, specialized blends for mental tasks, or innovative ways to incorporate oils into daily life.

In this final chapter, we will explore where essential oils may head in the coming years. We will look at scientific studies, technology breakthroughs, and market shifts that can shape how people use and think about these potent plant extracts.

20.2 Scientific Research on Essential Oils

1. **Clinical Studies on Efficacy**
    - While anecdotal experiences are common, more rigorous trials are taking place. For instance, small studies look at how certain oils might ease mild stress or support sleep quality.
    - Some researchers test antimicrobial properties or compare oils to conventional treatments in controlled settings.
2. **Phytochemical Analysis**
    - Gas Chromatography–Mass Spectrometry (GC-MS) and other tools help scientists map the molecules inside each oil.
    - Understanding compounds like linalool, limonene, or eugenol can help explain possible effects and safety concerns.
3. **Precision Blending**

- A few labs examine synergy between compounds. If one compound seems beneficial, does combining it with another enhance or reduce the effect?
- This can lead to more targeted formulations.

4. **Evidence-Based Guidelines**
    - As data grows, professional bodies may set clearer guidelines for use, recommended dilutions, or cautions for vulnerable groups.
    - This might reduce confusion and unify best practices across different brands and countries.

Scientific breakthroughs can bring new credibility to essential oils, or they might highlight limitations. Either way, deeper knowledge can help practitioners and consumers make informed decisions.

20.3 Technology and Innovation

1. **Smart Diffusers**
    - Some devices now connect to Wi-Fi or apps, letting you set schedules or combine scent cartridges. You can program a morning wake-up blend or an evening relaxation setting.
    - Future models might adjust fragrance levels based on room size or air quality sensors.
2. **Ultrasonic vs. Nebulizing**
    - Different diffuser methods can impact how strongly the aroma fills the space. Nebulizing diffusers do not use water, so they might deliver a more concentrated scent.
    - We might see improvements in diffuser efficiency, noise reduction, or safety features (like auto-off timers).
3. **Encapsulation Techniques**
    - Companies explore ways to embed essential oils in microcapsules for gradual release over time. This could be used in fabrics, car interiors, or building materials.
    - Imagine a couch fabric that slowly releases lavender aroma when pressure is applied, or a pillow that helps maintain a mild scent all night.
4. **Biotechnology in Production**

- Researchers are looking at ways to produce certain aromatic compounds using microorganisms, reducing the need to harvest large amounts of plants.
- This can lessen environmental impact for rare oils, but also raises questions about what qualifies as "natural."

20.4 Sustainability and Ethical Concerns

1. **Overharvesting Threats**
    - Popular oils like frankincense or sandalwood can face ecological pressure if wild populations are taken too aggressively.
    - Groups push for replanting initiatives, controlled harvests, or synthetic equivalents to reduce strain on wild sources.
2. **Fair Wages for Farmers**
    - In some regions, small-scale farmers who grow or harvest plants for essential oils earn little. Fair trade programs aim to give them a better share.
    - Ethical brands highlight these partnerships as a selling point.
3. **Sustainable Packaging**
    - More brands switch to eco-friendlier packaging, cutting plastic or using recycled materials.
    - Some offer refill options to reduce waste.
4. **Regenerative Agriculture**
    - Instead of just organic methods, some farms explore regenerative practices that improve soil health, biodiversity, and water retention.
    - Essential oil crops like lavender or clary sage can fit well into rotational farming systems.

Consumers are increasingly aware of these matters. A brand showing genuine care for the environment and local communities might gain more trust in future.

20.5 New Uses and Product Categories

1. **Aromatherapy in Wearables**
    - Small jewelry items (like lockets or bracelets) can hold a blotter with a drop of oil for personal inhalation on the go.
    - Tech-enabled wearables might control the release of scent in small pulses, though this is still niche.
2. **Public Spaces and Offices**
    - Some offices or retail stores diffuse mild scents to influence mood or reduce stress.
    - Future building designs might integrate scent systems into ventilation, although safety for all employees (including those sensitive to fragrances) remains a topic of debate.
3. **Food and Beverage Innovations**
    - More chefs experiment with safe culinary-grade essential oils.
    - Bakeries or specialty drink shops might craft signature items with a drop of peppermint, basil, or lemon oil, as we discussed. Strict care about dosage is vital.
4. **Veterinary and Pet Products**
    - Ongoing attempts exist to produce truly pet-safe essential oil solutions. But it remains an area with many cautions.
    - If research identifies safe formulas, we might see more veterinarian-approved lines for mild pet issues.

20.6 Professional Aromatherapy Growth

Aromatherapy is not just a hobby. More people seek formal training:

1. **Accredited Courses**
    - Schools and online programs now provide structured certificates or diplomas.
    - Students learn anatomy, physiology, chemistry, blending, and business skills.
2. **Clinical Aromatherapy**

- Hospitals or clinics sometimes welcome certified aromatherapists to offer mild supportive therapies for stress or comfort.
- More research might lead to official guidelines on how staff can safely use essential oils in medical settings.

3. **Specialized Fields**
   - Some professionals focus on palliative care, mental wellness, or sports therapy with essential oils as a tool.
   - Over time, we might see specific titles like "aromatherapy consultant for mental health support," though that requires clear boundaries and training.

As formal education advances, the profession may standardize, weeding out misinformation or unsafe practices.

20.7 Consumer Demand for Customization

1. **Personalized Blends**
   - Some consumers want custom scents tailored to their preferences or emotional needs.
   - Apps might guide them to select oils based on a quiz about mood or scent likes.
   - Small businesses offering custom blend consultations may see growth.
2. **DNA or Genetic-Based Approaches**
   - While still speculative, a few companies talk about matching scents or products to someone's unique biology.
   - This raises questions about privacy, cost, and scientific validity.
3. **Aromatherapy Subscriptions**
   - A monthly or quarterly box with curated blends or single oils for various themes (stress relief, immunity, seasonal changes) remains popular.
   - Subscribers enjoy trying new scents regularly without the hassle of picking each product individually.

20.8 Medical Community's Evolving Stance

Opinions vary within the medical world. Some doctors remain skeptical, pointing to the lack of large-scale randomized trials. Others see potential benefits if used responsibly:

- **Integrative Clinics**: Certain clinics combine mainstream medicine with complementary therapies, including essential oils for minor stress or comfort.
- **Safety Protocols**: The presence of clear instructions on dilution, possible interactions with medication, or restricted uses for pregnant individuals might help doctors feel more comfortable suggesting certain products.
- **Continuing Education**: Health professionals might attend short aromatherapy courses to learn how to advise patients on safe usage. This can reduce misuse or misunderstandings.

If more robust evidence emerges, we may see formal guidelines from medical associations on certain uses, such as stress relief or mild discomfort.

20.9 Genetic Research on Plant Varieties

Farmers and scientists are breeding or discovering plant strains that yield higher amounts of desired compounds. For instance:

- **Lavender Strains**
    - Some farms specialize in types high in linalool (believed to have calming properties).
    - This can produce more consistent essential oils with predictable scents.
- **Disease-Resistant Crops**
    - If a fungus threatens certain crops (like rose or geranium), new strains might be developed for resilience.
    - This stabilizes supply and possibly lowers the cost.
- **Heirloom vs. Hybrid**

- There is still debate about preserving traditional plant varieties vs. creating hybrids for commercial yield.
- Some customers prefer heirloom plants for their unique aroma, even if the yield is smaller.

20.10 Rare Applications

Some lesser-known uses for essential oils might expand:

1. **Natural Pest Management**
   - Farms sometimes spray diluted essential oils to repel insects from crops.
   - Homeowners use them to deter ants or spiders, though caution is necessary for pets and children.
2. **Textile Fragrances**
   - Infusing clothing or linens with microencapsulated oils that release scent over time. This is seen in some bedding or workout gear, though large-scale usage is still niche.
3. **Emotional and Cognitive Support**
   - Research is looking into how certain scents might stimulate memory recall (in Alzheimer's patients, for example).
   - Another area is studying if peppermint or rosemary aroma can help with mild mental alertness in specific tasks.

While each new use must be tested for safety and effectiveness, the curiosity around essential oils remains high.

20.11 Debates and Future Outlook

There are tensions in the essential oil community:

- **Purity vs. Synthetics**: Some want only pure, unaltered oils from plants, while others see value in lab-made versions for cost or sustainability reasons.

- **Claims and Reality**: Overstated health benefits can damage credibility. Some businesses might pivot to more modest, evidence-based statements.
- **Market Saturation**: As more sellers enter, competition can lead to pricing wars. High-quality producers might rely on branding and direct farm relationships to stand out.
- **Regulation**: Governments could tighten rules on labeling or marketing. This can protect consumers but also raise business costs.

Still, essential oils are likely to keep a solid place in wellness, beauty, and home care for many years, especially as society leans toward natural solutions.

20.12 Ongoing Safety Discussions

Even with future developments, safety will remain a top concern:

- **Proper Dilutions**: More standard charts or guidelines might become mainstream, so fewer people apply undiluted oils or accidentally ingest them.
- **Sensitive Populations**: Greater emphasis on warnings for pregnant women, children, older adults, or those with health conditions.
- **Public Awareness**: As usage grows, hopefully education about possible risks (like skin sensitization, phototoxicity, or pet hazards) spreads too.

Well-informed consumers and more consistent product labeling can reduce accidental misuse.

20.13 Role of Digital Platforms

Technology is reshaping how we learn about and buy oils:

- **Online Communities**

- People share recipes, tips, and experiences on social media or forums.
- However, misinformation also spreads easily. Credible sources or moderated groups help keep facts straight.
- **E-Commerce**
  - Automated shipping, subscription services, and personalized recommendations are common.
  - Some sites offer "oil finder" tools based on a user's mood or need, though these are often marketing-driven.
- **Augmented Reality (AR)**
  - A future possibility: Virtual smell apps are not yet feasible, but AR or VR might let you explore distilleries or see a 3D plant model while reading about its oil. This remains mostly conceptual.

20.14 Potential Crossovers with Other Fields

1. **Cosmetic and Dermatology Research**
   - Essential oils could be studied more in the context of skincare, for mild acne or scalp health.
   - Dermatologists might identify which oils are less likely to cause irritation.
2. **Nutraceuticals**
   - Some food scientists investigate safe microdoses of essential oils in functional beverages or supplements.
   - This is a controversial area, and strict regulation often applies.
3. **Mental Health Interventions**
   - Coupling scents with mindfulness or breathing techniques is a growing trend.
   - More data might show whether certain oils truly support relaxation or if the effect is mostly about the ritual and environment.
4. **Robotics and Automation**
   - Factories that produce or bottle essential oils might adopt more automation for precise measurements.

- This can reduce errors or contamination in large-scale production.

20.15 Rare Insights on Future Sustainability

- **Multi-Crop Plantations**: Instead of large monocultures of one aromatic plant, some farmers rotate or interplant species. This can improve soil health and reduce pests naturally.
- **Waste Reduction**: Distillation can leave plant residues. Some innovators turn that residue into compost, animal feed, or biomass energy.
- **Corporate Responsibility**: Big companies that buy essential oils might set strict rules on labor conditions, pesticide usage, or reforestation. They might also sponsor local communities to build schools or infrastructure in exchange for stable supplies.

Such practices could elevate the entire sector's image and actual impact on nature and people.

20.16 Advocacy and Consumer Movements

In the age of social media, advocacy groups can sway popular opinion:

1. **Calls for Label Clarity**
   - People want to know if something is truly pure or if it contains additives. Some push for more uniform labeling laws.
2. **Anti-Greenwashing**
   - Watchdogs highlight companies that claim to be "all-natural" but have hidden synthetic components or unethical sourcing.
3. **Organized Aromatherapists**
   - Professional groups might unify to publish best practice guidelines, clarifying safe use and disclaimers.

Public awareness can force companies to maintain higher standards or face backlash.

20.17 Educational Shifts

Future generations might learn about essential oils in new ways:

- **School Programs**: Some science classes might introduce basic distillation or the concept of plant-based extracts.
- **Online Academies**: More specialized or advanced online courses with thorough curriculums can certify students in advanced topics like in-depth chemistry or complex blending.
- **Mentorship**: Experienced aromatherapists might mentor younger entrepreneurs, passing on knowledge about sourcing and blending.

This can reshape how the next wave of enthusiasts approaches essential oils.

20.18 Encouraging Responsible Use

As essential oils remain popular, industry players and professionals can:

- **Offer Clear Usage Guides**: Simplify instructions (like "1 drop per teaspoon of carrier oil for adults").
- **Highlight Warnings**: Remind buyers about phototoxic oils or child safety.
- **Promote Patch Tests**: Make this common knowledge, not an afterthought.
- **Contribute to Valid Research**: Companies can sponsor academic studies or donate materials for clinical trials.

Such efforts might reduce accidents and build overall trust.

20.19 Personal Reflection for the Future

For those who love essential oils:

- **Stay Curious**: Keep reading new findings. The science is always evolving.
- **Adapt Your Practices**: If new data suggests different dilutions, change your approach.
- **Respect Nature**: Remember these oils come from plants that need healthy ecosystems. Support companies that care about the environment.
- **Protect Others**: Help friends or family who are new to essential oils learn safe methods.

By doing this, you remain a responsible participant in a field that blends tradition with modern discovery.

20.20 Conclusion

Essential oils will likely stay part of many routines, from personal care to household tasks, for years to come. Ongoing research can shine light on which practices are truly effective and which are unproven lore. Technological improvements may refine how we produce, store, and apply these oils, and careful sustainability efforts can protect both plants and farming communities.

At the same time, it remains important to approach essential oils with realistic expectations and a respect for their potency. Whether you are an enthusiast, a business owner, or a health professional, staying informed about future trends and research can help you use and recommend essential oils more wisely. The potential for new formulations, advanced diffusers, and evidence-based applications is significant, but safety, integrity, and environmental stewardship must guide every step.

In closing, essential oils have come far from ancient distillation pots to modern labs and apps. As the science develops and the market changes, a balance between tradition and innovation can keep this field vibrant. By following strong principles and continuing to learn, you can make the most of these fragrant gifts, responsibly and creatively, in the years ahead.

www.ingramcontent.com/pod-product-compliance
Lightning Source LLC
LaVergne TN
LVHW012104070526
838202LV00056B/5616